REVERSING
FIBROMYALGIA

How to Treat and Overcome
Fibromyalgia and Other
Arthritis-Related Diseases

REVERSING
FIBROMYALGIA

How to Treat and Overcome Fibromyalgia and Other Arthritis-Related Diseases

DR. JOE M. ELROD

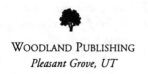

WOODLAND PUBLISHING
Pleasant Grove, UT

CONTENTS

Note from the Author

As an exercise physiologist specializing in heart disease, high blood pressure, diabetes, and other systemic conditions, I began to come in contact with the term fibromyalgia on a rather frequent basis beginning about five or six years ago. As I continued to work as a college professor and as a consultant with various organizations in the area of health and wellness, I was continually confronted with people who thought they might have fibromyalgia and asking advice as to what they should do about it and therefore I became very frustrated as I began to look for answers, research the area, only to find there were no books available, there was very little information in the libraries to be found anywhere. Therefore, I became keenly interested in finding something that would slow down or reverse the progression of the disease, rather than just to relieve pain.

Seemingly the only approaches taken in treating fibromyalgia were the use on nonsteroidal anti-inflammatory drugs along with acetaminophen and antidepressants to help relieve pain and to try to help fibromyalgia sufferer's sleep. Physicians seemed initially to believe that these drugs would slow the progression of fibromyalgia and eventually help the patients improve over time. However, over the years experience and research has shown that this is probably not the case.

Fortunately for about ten years or so I had been conducting research in the areas of vitamins, minerals, and herbs and had a bevy of information on positive results in the use of these with various people from around the world. Excited to learn whether or not we could be successful by utilizing many of the various combinations of natural supplements with fibromyalgia and arthritic victims, I cautiously began to design programs, giving them to clients and people with whom I was working directly. I also began to utilize my former training and background in the areas of exercise, nutrition, and stress management to develop a complete, natural, healing program for these people. I have been using various aspects of the program design in this book for more than three years now and the people with whom I have worked have experience tremendous results. We are most excited about the potential of the future because in many, many cases we have found the symptoms and conditions of fibromyalgia and arthritis were totally reversed.

As you read this book and attempt to make a decision along with your physician as to whether to follow this program, you should consider the following:

• Fibromyalgia impacts every individual in a different way and no two people will respond the same way to the treatment regimens or programs that have been designed within this book.

• This program is very safe and can be a very effective treatment alternative and you can expect very little if any side effects because of its all natural nature. Even if your fibromyalgia is in the very severe stages, you can still expect to receive dramatic relief; it may just take a bit longer than a person in the earlier stages.

• Although this program has not worked 100 percent for all individuals who have tried it, you can fully expect to make progress and even get well with a full commitment to this program. Remember, the program in this book is designed to treat the basic cause of your condition and not simply mask the symptoms to relieve pain temporarily.

We now know that fibromyalgia can be more than managed—it can be reversed. People simply do not have to accept the bleak prognosis that they will have to live with it the rest of their life. May the guidelines in this book provide you with the information and impetus to overcome your condition and live a healthier, happier life.

CHAPTER 1

What Is
Fibromyalgia?

Fibromyalgia is a common clinical syndrome of generalized musculoskeletal pain, stiffness, and chronic aching characterized by reproducible tenderness on palpation of specific anatomical sites generally referred to as tender points. This condition is considered primary when not associated with a systemic cause such as trauma, cancer, thyroid disease, and pathologies of rheumatic arthritis or connective tissues. Fibromyalgia is more common in middle-aged women between the ages of 30 and 50 years. It is now recognized as one of the most common rheumatic complaints with clinical prevalence and accounts for 10 to 30 percent of all rheumatology consultations in North America (Bennett, 1989).

The name fibromyalgia has largely replaced the term *fibrositis* which was once used to describe this disorder. The "itis" means inflammation of a bodily process that can result in pain, swelling, warmth, stiffness, and redness. Earlier research described this condition as inflammation in muscles, but during the past fifty years research has all but proven that inflammation is not a significant part of fibromyalgia.

A Muscular/Soft Tissue Condition

Fibromyalgia is really a form of muscular and "soft tissue" rheumatism, rather than arthritis of the joints. The word rheumatism refers to the pain and stiffness associated with arthritis and related disorders of the joints, muscles, and bones. Fibromyalgia mainly affects muscles and their attachments to bones, especially in the areas of muscle/tendon junctions (Bennett, 1989). The name "fibromyalgia" means pain in the muscles and in the fibrous connective tissues. This condition is referred to as a syndrome because it is a set of signs and symptoms that occur together. (A sign is what the physician or health professional finds on examination; a symptom is what the person reports to the health care professional or the doctor.)

PRIMARY SYMPTOMS OF FIBROMYALGIA

- Tenderness of at least 11 of 18 specific anatomical sites (see Figure 1 later in this chapter for specific diagnosis information.)
- Chronic aching
- Stiffness
- Sleep disturbances
- Pain
- Fatigue
- Anxiety
- Depression
- Chronic Fatigue
- Gastrointestinal disturbances
- Subjective soft tissue swelling
- Cardiovascular problems (dizziness, palpitations)

Most patients with fibromyalgia syndrome state that they literally ache all over. They describe their muscles as feeling as if they have been pulled, torn, or overworked, sometimes twitching and at other times burning. The severity of symptoms will fluctuate tremendously from one person to the next. Fibromyalgia syndrome sometimes resembles a post-viral state, which is one of the reasons some experts and researchers in the field believe that fibromyalgia syndrome and chronic fatigue syndrome are one and the same (Goldenberg, 1990). According to Wolfe (1993), the only thing that differentiates between the two is the degree of pain.

Family, friends and work associates of patients with fibromyalgia very often have a difficult time understanding their condition because blood tests and x-rays reveal no physical evidence. I suggest that they might think back to the last time they had the flu, when every muscle in the body ached and they felt totally drained of energy. This might help them understand what it feels like to have fibromyalgia.

Who Is Affected?

Seven to ten million Americans suffer from fibromyalgia. It is seen in all age groups from young children to old age, although in most patients, the problem begins in their twenties or thirties. Fibromyalgia affects women much more than men in an approximate ratio of 50 to 1 (Pellgrino, 1989).

Fibromyalgia is not Arthritis

Fibromyalgia syndrome patients have widespread body pain that originates from their muscles. Some fibromyalgia patients feel that pain is focused in their joints, similar to arthritis, but extensive studies have shown that fibromyalgia patients do not have arthritis (Campbell, 1983). Although many fibromyalgia patients are aware of pain when they are resting, it is most noticeable when they use their muscles, particularly in exercise. Their discomfort can be so severe it may significantly limit their ability to lead a full life. At times patients find themselves unable to work in their chosen professions and may have difficulty performing everyday tasks. As a consequence of muscle pain, many fibromyalgia patients severely limit their activities and exercise (McCain, 1988). This results in their becoming physically unfit which eventually makes their fibromyalgia symptoms worse. (See the chapter 6 on exercise for the appropriate "whys and hows" for health and recovery.)

In addition to generally widespread bodily pain, other common symptoms include a decreased sense of energy, disturbances of sleep, and varying degrees of anxiety and depression relating to the patient's changed physical status. Furthermore, certain other medical conditions are commonly associated with fibromyalgia, such as tension headaches, migraine headaches, irritable bowel syndrome, irritable bladder syndrome, premenstrual tension syndrome, cold intolerance, and restless leg syndrome. This combination of pain and multiple other symptoms often lead physicians and other professionals to pursue a sometimes confusing but extensive course of investigations (Hobson, 1968).

One of the more devastating symptoms of fibromyalgia syndrome is a sleep disorder. During sleep we usually have periods when we stop moving and go into a deep, very restful, recharging sleep (level 4). Unfortunately, in fibromyalgia, the pain of the muscles and connective tissue makes it impossible to lie in one position for an extended period of time. As a result the patient is continually brought back into light sleep. Fibromyalgia patients simply do not experience the deep stages of sleep that allow for complete rest. Even when they sleep for eight hours each night they can awaken tired each morning (May, 1993).

How Is It Diagnosed?

When trying to diagnose fibromyalgia, normal laboratory testing will reveal absolutely nothing. In other words, blood tests or x-rays are of no value. This fact initially led physicians to consider the problem described by these patients to be "in their heads," a form of masked depression or hypochondriasis. However, later research involving extensive physiological tests has shown that these impressions were untrue or unfounded (Goldenberg, 1989).

A diagnosis of fibromyalgia by health professionals or physicians is based on taking a careful personal or family history and by pinpointing tender areas in specific locations of muscle throughout the body. One of the general guidelines followed for diagnostic criteria is a demonstration of widespread pain in all four quadrants of the body for a minimum duration of three months and sensitivity in 11 of the 18 tender point sites. (See Figure 1 on next page.)

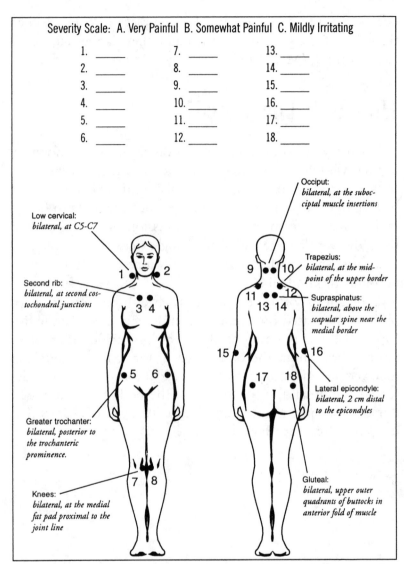

Severity Scale: A. Very Painful B. Somewhat Painful C. Mildly Irritating

1. _____	7. _____	13. _____
2. _____	8. _____	14. _____
3. _____	9. _____	15. _____
4. _____	10. _____	16. _____
5. _____	11. _____	17. _____
6. _____	12. _____	18. _____

Occiput:
bilateral, at the suboccipital muscle insertions

Low cervical:
bilateral, at C5-C7

Trapezius:
bilateral, at the midpoint of the upper border

Second rib:
bilateral, at second costochondral junctions

Supraspinatus:
bilateral, above the scapular spine near the medial border

Lateral epicondyle:
bilateral, 2 cm distal to the epicondyles

Greater trochanter:
bilateral, posterior to the trochanteric prominence.

Gluteal:
bilateral, upper outer quadrants of buttocks in anterior fold of muscle

Knees:
bilateral, at the medial fat pad proximal to the joint line

Figure 1: *Tender Points for Diagnosis of Fibromyalgia*
(American College of Rheumatology, 1990)

Evidence to show that we are making progress with fibromyalgia diagnosis was revealed in a 1990 multi-center criteria study published in the February 1990 issue of *Arthritis and Rheumatism*. In an experimental group of 558 patients, 265 were classified with fibromyalgia syndrome. The control group were not your typical healthy individuals. All the age and sex matched patients exhibited neck pain, low back pain, trauma related pain syndromes, tendonitis, rheumatoid arthritis, lupus, and other painful disorders. Each patient had some symptoms which are similar to fibromyalgia syndrome. Trained examiners hand-picked those with fibromyalgia out of the chronically ill melting pot with an accuracy rate of 88 percent (Wolfe, 1990).

Although there are no specific diagnostic lab tests for fibromyalgia, there is good reason to have medical tests done. Primarily, this would be done to rule out several conditions that could be confused with fibromyalgia and help to avoid a misdiagnosis. For instance, an SED rate should be done on older patients to rule out polymyalgia rheumatica. Systemic conditions such as lupus and hypothyroidism should also be checked for and ruled out.

Finally, the only difference between the fibromyalgia and chronic fatigue syndrome patient is the degree of pain (Goldenberg, 1990; Buchwald, 1987). About 75 percent of patients diagnosed with chronic fatigue syndrome will meet the criteria of fibromyalgia syndrome (Buchwald, 1987). Experts deem it unlikely that these two conditions are separate disease processes. According to Dr. David A. Nye, the current syndrome definition is all we have, based on numerous studies that have been done. At some point, once we know more about the true etiology (cause), an etiologic diagnosis rather than a syndromic diagnosis can be made.

ETIOLOGY: WHAT CAUSES FIBROMYALGIA?

It is reported in medical literature that a single, exact cause of fibromyalgia is at this time unknown. However, there are many events that could cause or that are "thought" to precipitate the onset of fibromyalgia. For example, close to 100 percent of the fibromyalgia victims I have personally worked with have all experienced a long period of undue stress or emotional trauma—whether it be an automobile accident, divorce, a long illness, growing up in a dysfunctional family, experiencing abuse as a child, or some other type of trauma. It is reported that these triggering events probably do not cause fibromyalgia, but rather they awaken or provoke an underlying physiological abnormality that is already existent. One theory is that physical or emotional trauma can precipitate fibromyalgia in a number of ways. For example, a physical trauma such as having an infection or flu can lead to certain hormonal or chemical changes that promote pain and disturbed sleep. Also, those with fibromyalgia may become inactive, causing them to feel anxious about their health and further aggravating the disorder. Recent studies have shown that in fibromyalgia the muscles are especially vulnerable to decreased circulation and minor injury (Bennett, 1989).

What About the Pain?

The pain associated with fibromyalgia syndrome is the most prominent symptom of the condition. Patients describe the pain as deep, burning, throbbing, and stabbing. The pain is generally felt throughout the body, although it starts in one region such as the neck and shoulders, and then seems to spread over time to other parts of the body. The pain will often vary, depending on the time of day, activity level, the weather, sleep patterns, and interruptions in lifestyle. Most fibromyalgia patients report that some degree of pain is consistently present. Most often the pain and stiffness are worse in the early morning and are worse in muscles that are used repetitively. In many cases physicians are not familiar with evaluation of the tender points, but rheumatologists (specialists in arthritis and rheumatism) will usually know when and how to perform the examination to diagnose fibromyalgia syndrome.

Though there appears to be no specific diagnostic test available, recent research suggests that people with fibromyalgia are physiologically different. Dr. Laurence Bradley, professor of medicine at the Division of Clinical Immunology and Rheumatology at the University of Alabama in Birmingham, is leading a scientific team in this investigation. The team discovered that the cerebral spinal fluid in those with fibromyalgia contains more substance P, a neuropeptide that serves as a peripheral pain neurotransmitter that carries pain signals. High levels means that it is more likely that pain is perceived. Dr. Bradley says, "It's almost like those with fibromyalgia have a pain filter that's not working well."

The exact initial trigger for the faulty filters, the mineral deficiencies, the disrupted energy production cycles, and the disrupted sleep patterns are largely specifically unknown. However, the more prominent theory appears to be severe stress coupled with emotionally traumatic experiences, especially over extended periods of time. Another study in 1994 revealed similar findings and supported the fact of a peripheral origin for fibromyalgia pain (Russell, 1996). Crofford (1994) and Moldofsky (1995) have identified similar neuroendocrine abnormalities in other studies which help to continue to form the basis of the etiology of fibromyalgia.

It has also been suggested that fibromyalgia pain is related to microtrauma in deconditioned muscles, and that the right kind of exercise is beneficial for reconditioning these muscles (see exercise chapter) (Bennett, 1989). The tender areas of fibromyalgia, or "trigger points" as they are sometimes referred to, are similar in location to sore and tender areas in other common muscle and bone pain disorders such as tennis elbow and trochanteric bursitis (inflammation of the outer side of the hip). Those with fibromyalgia very often are not aware of the exact location or even the presence of many of the trigger points until they are specifically examined by a health professional or physician.

Fatigue and Sleep Disorders

The fatigue associated with fibromyalgia has been described as "brain fatigue" in which people feel totally drained of energy. The fatigue symptom can be mild in some and incapacitating in others. Ninety percent of those with fibromyalgia describe moderate or severe fatigue similar to the exhaustion experienced with the flu. Very often fatigue is more of a problem than pain. Many patients state that they feel as if their arms are tied to concrete blocks and they have great difficulty concentrating. Most will generally have difficulty sleeping and will wake up feeling very tired.

Scientific studies (Campbell, 1983) indicate that most people with fibromyalgia have an abnormal sleep pattern marked by interruptions in their deep sleep. In one study done in a sleep lab, researchers found that those with fibromyalgia could fall asleep without much difficulty at all. However, their deep sleep (stage 4) level was constantly interrupted by bursts of awake-like brain activity. This coincides with the fact that low levels of growth hormone, important in maintaining good muscles and other soft tissue health, have been found in people with fibromyalgia. This hormone is produced almost exclusively in deep sleep, and its production is increased by exercise.

Physicians typically do not have to order expensive sleep lab tests to determine if one has had disturbed sleep. If the individual wakes up feeling as though they have been awake all night, doctors refer to this as unrefreshed sleep. It is reasonable for a physician or a health professional to assume or to classify this as a sleep disorder. Many fibromyalgia sufferers have an associated deep sleep disorder called Alpha-EEG Anomaly. Most people diagnosed with chronic fatigue syndrome have the same Alpha-EEG sleep pattern. Also, some fibromyalgia diagnosed patients have been found to have other sleep disorders, such as sleep apnea, sleep myocoonus (night time jerking of the arms and legs), restless leg syndrome, and bruxism (teeth grinding). Note: It has been determined that the sleep pattern for clinically depressed patients is distinctly different from that found in those with fibromyalgia or chronic fatigue syndrome (Moldofsky, 1975). Other common symptoms of fibromyalgia are:

- Chest pain
- Morning stiffness
- Cognitive or memory impairment
- Premenstrual syndrome and painful periods
- Tingling sensations and numbness in limbs
- Irritable bladder
- Muscular twitching
- The feeling of swollen extremities or subjective soft tissue swelling
- Skin sensitivities

- Dry eyes and mouth
- Frequent changes in eye prescription
- Dizziness and impaired coordination.

Suspected Culprits: Stress and Trauma

Another theory currently being evaluated as a possible cause of fibromyalgia is the body's response to stress and trauma. Researchers are trying to determine if the autonomic nervous system works properly under such conditions. Long periods of undue stress and emotional disruption appear to be the underlying cause of energy compound deficiencies. Over long periods, trauma interrupts the natural physiological process of ATP (energy) production. Along with prolonged stress and trauma, poor diet, lack of exercise, and lack of the proper nutrients and supplements (vitamins, minerals, and antioxidants) will begin to weaken the immune system to the point that the body will yield to the onset of fibromyalgia.

There are other theories about the causes of fibromyalgia that pertain to neurotransmitter regulation (particularly serotonin and norepinephrine), immune system function, sleep physiology, and hormonal control that are under investigation (Baldessarini, 1985). Additionally, modern brain imaging techniques are being used to explore various aspects of brain function.

Vitamin and Mineral Deficiencies

THE B-COMPLEX VITAMINS

Thiamin (B1), riboflavin (B2), and pyridoxine (B6)* are essential for electron transport in the respiratory system. All three vitamins require a magnesium-dependent phosphate transferring action to become biologically active. When there is a magnesium deficiency there is a breakdown in the body's energy production process (See Table 1). The five ingredients required for the synthesis of ATP—required for energy and movement—and some of the conditions postulated to cause a deficiency of each ingredient are shown in the table. Magnesium is one of the key ingredients of the formula and it has been found that almost all fibromyalgia patients have a magnesium deficiency. Most migraine headache victims will also demonstrate a magnesium deficiency.

Requirements	Primary Sources	Intramitochondrial Conditions Postulated to Cause a Deficiency
oxygen	cardiopulmonary	hypoxia, malate deficiency, magnesium deficiency
magnesium	food	excess aluminum, excess calcium
substrate	food	severe malnutrition, malate def.
ADP	ATP	phosphate def., magn. def.
inorganic phosphate	food	mang. def., excess calcium, malate deficiency, excess aluminum
capacity of the respiratory chain	food/genetics	vitamins B1, B2, B6 essential for the electron transport system in the respiratory chain. These three vitamins require a magnesium dependent phosphate transfer reaction to become biologically active.
mitochondrial membrane integrity	food/genetics	magnesium deficiency causes mitochondrial swelling, increased membrane permeability and uncoupling of oxidative phosphorylation.

Table 1. *Requirements for optimal synthesis of ATP by intact respiring mitochondria: critical roles of malate and magnesium.* (Reprinted from the *Journal of Nutritional Medicine*, Vol. 3, 1992)

The following list of events or conditions commonly contribute to the onset of fibromyalgia:

- Traumatic emotional experience
- Stress and/or depression
- Magnesium, phosphate, substrate, and oxygen deficiencies
- Biological disruption of energy production
- Chronic fatigue
- Low levels of growth hormone
- Disruption of deep sleep

THE ROLE OF MAGNESIUM IN ENERGY PRODUCTION

Some current research is now indicating that fibromyalgia sufferers are deficient in certain compounds that are required for the production of energy physiologically. The presence of magnesium, substrate oxygen, and phosphates are essential for energy production. Concentrations at very high levels are required for healthy cellular respiration and the concomitant production of biological energy. On the other hand, deficiencies in these substances can seriously impede the Krebs cycle (human energy cycle), causing a reduction of the ability of the body to utilize oxygen for muscle energy. This current research has definitely confirmed that a deficiency of the above factors can very clearly lead to the symptoms of fatigue and depression in the fibromyalgia victims.

Also, new research suggests that magnesium, being one of the most crucial elements for ATP synthesis, is usually below normal range when measured in fibromyalgia patients. The Krebs cycle) is a magnesium dependent mechanism and even a slight deficiency of the element will severely impair its optimal function.

WHAT ABOUT ALUMINUM?

It is now known that magnesium is needed to help the body block toxic effects of aluminum; therefore, aluminum toxicity may play a role in symptoms experienced by magnesium deficient fibromyalgia patients (Weintraub, 1997). Aluminum inhibits glycolysis (the production of energy) and oxidative phosphorylation. Additionally, due to its high affinity for phosphate groups, aluminum blocks the absorption and utilization of phosphates that are critical to the creation of energy. The possible effects of aluminum toxicity on fibromyalgia sufferers needs to be acknowledged and addressed.

MAGNESIUM AND MALIC ACID– A HELPFUL COMBINATION

Since aluminum has been identified as a toxic metal leading to major metabolic disturbances, researchers have carefully studied means of eliminating it from the body's vital organs. It has been discovered that proper amounts of magnesium, along with supplemental malic acid, can act as a most potent aluminum detoxifier and are especially effective at decreasing aluminum toxicity in the vital organs of the body, especially the brain. Malic acid is effective because it has been shown to significantly increase the fecal and urinary secretion of aluminum, reducing the concentration of the metal found in the internal organs, tissues, and the brain (Weintraub, 1997).

A recently published research study shows the combined effects of malic acid and magnesium on fibromyalgia patients. Fifteen patients between the ages of 32 and 60 were used in an open clinical setting where oral magnesium and malic acid preparations were ingested for a period of four to eight weeks. The patients ingested 1200-2400 milligrams of malic acid with 30-600 milligrams of magnesium. The results of the study are encouraging as all patients reported significant relief of pain within just 48 hours of treatment. Results of studies such as this one gives us continuous hope for the fibromyalgia patient through nutritional and supplemental treatment (Abraham, 1992).

MANGANESE–A CRITICAL SUPPLEMENT

Recent studies have investigated the link between chronic fatigue syndrome and fibromyalgia syndrome, specifically why fatigue is one of the most prominent features in both syndromes. It may have something to do with manganese dependent neuroendocrine changes, especially along the hypothalamic-pituitary-thyroid axis. The cycle begins with hypothalamic production of thyrotropin-releasing hormones (TRH). TRH stimulates the pituitary gland to produce thyroid stimulating hormones (TSH) which in turn stimulates thyroid production of thyroxin.

This is critical simply because thyroxin regulates the metabolic rate. Since fatigue is one of the primary conditions of both fibromyalgia and chronic fatigue victims, hypometabolism due to secondary hypothyroidism fits very nicely into the hypothesis. Manganese directly influences the metabolic rate through its involvement in this hypothalamic-pituitary-thyroid axis and may therefore be a helpful trace mineral supplement for both fibromyalgia and chronic fatigue victims.

In view of the above, it would make good sense for those with fibromyalgia to employ nutritional supplementation of magnesium, malic acid, and manganese for the production of energy, for aluminum detoxification, and to enhance metabolism in the recovery and return to general health and well-being.

A Fallacy: Fibromyalgia Cannot Be Cured

The chronic problems of musculoskeletal pain and fatigue are common afflictions that most doctors believe are incurable. Generally, the patient is simply told that the pain is somewhat manageable through the use of drugs and therapy. This good news is that this is no longer true. The fibromyalgia cure has helped many fibromyalgia sufferers return to vibrant, productive health.

CHAPTER 2

Traditional Treatments of Fibromyalgia

The treatment of fibromyalgia has traditionally been geared toward using drugs to reduce pain and increase the quality of sleep. Sleep disorders that frequently occur in fibromyalgia patients are thought to be a major contributing factor to the symptoms of the condition. Traditionally, the medications that have been prescribed for fibromyalgia are those that boost the body's level of a neurotransmitter known as serotonin which modulates sleep, pain, and immune system function.

Overall, this method of treatment has not been very effective and, as a result, the treatment of fibromyalgia has been a frustrating venture historically for both patients and physicians (Nxrregaard et al., 1995). Other treatment modalities that have been utilized with fibromyalgia sufferers are trigger point injections with lidocaine, physical therapy, acupressure, acupuncture, and other techniques such as muscle relaxation, breathing exercises, osteopathic manipulation, and therapeutic massage.

General aerobic exercise programs have also been used since there has been increasing evidence that a regular program is very essential for fibromyalgia patients. In the past, physicians and health professionals have taken fibromyalgia victims off exercise because increased pain and fatigue can often result from repetitive movement and exertion, making exercise quite difficult. However, most of the people who do get into a proper exercise regimen experience worthwhile improvement and are very reluctant to give it up (McCain, 1988). (See more details on a proper exercise program in the Chapter 6.)

The major problem with drug treatments is that often, instead of getting to the source of the problem, they merely mask the symptoms. Another problem is that there are always side effects and very often these side effects can exacerbate the original problem and/or cause other problems that are as serious as the original condition. However, there are times when pain relievers may be very necessary and your physician will probably prescribe some (Jaeschke et al., 1991).

It is important that before taking any medication you understand what it is supposed to do and what the side effects may be. It is also helpful to explore the results of the various types of medications that are commonly used to treat fibromyalgia. I very strongly recommend that you follow your physician's advice when taking the medications prescribed for your condition. But it is my sincere hope that as you move toward a natural regimen and begin using nutrients such as magnesium, malic acid, coenzyme Q-10, and other antioxidants, phytonutrients, and bioflavonoids, that you will be able to reduce or lessen the need for drugs. As you proceed with your natural health and healing regimen, it will become easier.

DRUGS USED TO TREAT FIBROMYALGIA

This section looks at the various categories and specific drugs that have been used in traditional treatment of fibromyalgia, some of the problems associated with the drugs, and what can be expected based on the accumulated research and history of their use (Bennet, Goldenberg, and McCain).

Antidepressants

The reason nonaddictive antidepressant drugs are used is to assist the inducement of deep sleep. Medications that have been traditionally prescribed to boost the body's level of serotonin include amitriptyline, elavil, and clobenzaprine (flexeril). Other drugs that have often been prescribed are zanax (same as alprazalam), paxil, and klonopin. These medications have assisted in better sleep and provided for less discomfort, but the improvement does vary greatly from person to person. Beware of side effects such as dry mouth, daytime drowsiness, increased appetite, and constipation. Although these side effects are rarely severe, they can be disturbing and may limit the use of the drugs (Russell, 1991). It is also very important to avoid prescription tranquilizers and sleeping medications of the benzodiazepine group. While these may help or assist sleep, they suppress deep sleep and often make fibromyalgia symptoms worse. Finally, the routine use of sleeping pills such as valium, halcion, and restoril should be avoided as they impair the quality of deep sleep and can also be addictive.

Corticosteroids

Powerful drugs such as prednisone and cortisone are corticosteroids that are sometimes prescribed for severe pain. They are excellent at reducing such pain, but have some very serious side effects that put them in the "dangerous" category. Some of the side effects are thinning of the bones, impairment of wound healing, the risk of bone fracture, and depression of the immune system. When taken in large doses over long periods of time, corticosteroids can also cause osteoporosis, diabetes, hypertension, and have been reported to cause mental disturbances. These are some of the reasons that the NSAIDs were developed as alternatives to the corticosteroids (Calabro, 1992).

Corticosteroids can also cause serious problems in the nutrition area. They are a serious threat to decreasing the absorption of vitamin D, causing water retention and enhancing the rate of excretion of vitamin C, potassium, and zinc. When corticosteroids are prescribed, one would be wise to increase the supplementation of these nutrients. The good news is that, once you get well into your fibromyalgia cure regimen, the need for the prescription of these nutritionally disturbing medications will be lessened (Brooks and Day, 1991).

Acetaminophen and NSAIDs

Acetaminophen and NSAIDs (nonsteroidal anti-inflammatory drugs) are typically prescribed for similar reasons. Acetaminophen is sold under the trade names Tylenol, Liquiprin, and Datril. Some of the common nonsteroidal anti-inflammatory drugs are sold under the names of Motrin,

Advil, and aspirin. It is important to point out the differences between acetaminophen and NSAIDs. Both are prescribed as pain relievers and do an excellent job with relieving pain. However, acetaminophen is an analgesic and an antipyretic, which means that it relieves pain and lowers fever. Nonsteroidal anti-inflammatory drugs help reduce fever, fight pain, and remove inflammation. Some physicians will opt for prescribing acetaminophen since it is less expensive and has fewer side effects than the NSAIDs. However, do not be misled here because acetaminophen certainly has its own side effects (Gay, 1990).

According to Sandler (1989), acetaminophen is well tolerated and safe if taken in a standard dosage of below four grams per twenty-four hour period. However, if taken over a long period of time, acetaminophen carries the danger of a small but significant decrease in liver function, and possesses a possibility for harming the kidneys. In the *Harvard Health Letter*, Garnett (1995) suggests taking precautions with acetaminophen as studies and research show that it is probably the culprit in as many as 5,000 cases of kidney failure in the United States annually.

What About the NSAIDs?

Aspirin is by far the most popular and best known of the NSAIDs. It belongs to a class of drugs called salicylates used to treat osteoarthritis, various forms of rheumatism, and many other kinds of pain for more than 100 years. Small doses are typically used to treat pain while larger doses are generally prescribed to take care of inflammation. In the 1960s other NSAIDs such as indomethacin (indocin) were developed, followed by ibuprofen. The development of NSAIDs has continued and currently there are more than 100 different nonsteroidal anti-inflammatory drugs either on the market or under investigation for approval. Nonprescription, over-the-counter NSAIDs include Excedrin, Midol, Nuprin, Advil, and Motrin (Garnett, 1995).

Nonsteroidal anti-inflammatory drugs work primarily by impeding the production of prostaglandins, hormone substances in the body that enhance pain and inflammation responses. Prostaglandins, however, are also necessary in various body functions, such as the regulation of blood pressure, blood coagulation, the secretion of gastric juices in the stomach, and kidney regulation. As one would suspect, drugs that interfere with the negative actions of prostaglandins will also affect their positive purposes as well. This is the primary reason that NSAIDs have such a large number and serious side effects that interfere with bodily functions (Novak, 1995). Some of the common and potentially serious side effects are:

nausea	cramps
indigestion	diarrhea
constipation	sensitivity to sunlight
nervousness	confusion
drowsiness	headache
ulcers/stomach bleeding	high blood pressure
weight gain	swelling of hands/feet
urinary problems	sore throat/fever

Another side effect that is not so common is anaphylaxis, a rare, severe allergic reaction characterized by difficulty in breathing or swallowing, a swollen tongue, dizziness, fainting, hives, puffy eyelids, fast and irregular heartbeat or pulse, or a change in face color. This is an emergency situation; you should immediately seek help if you experience any of these signs after taking NSAIDs.

NSAIDs can be quite helpful when used on a short term basis to relieve pain, but can be very harmful when used over long periods because, though the pain is relieved, the underlying disease condition continues. Hendler (1992) points out that NSAIDs do notcure disease, so disease processes continue whether the patient feels the effects or not. In a five-year clinical study, Hodgkinson and Woolf (1979) reported that NSAIDs did not delay the progression of chronic pain diseases. In fact, they actually hastened their progress in some cases.

It is important to note that aspirin and other salicylates can have harmful side effects ranging from minor stomach upsets to life threatening hemorrhages. Also, as Dr. Theodosakis (1997) points out, while NSAIDs generally provide faster pain relief than natural supplements, the pain relief quickly plateaus and often diminishes with time. If pain and symptoms are severe, you may want to use pain relievers in conjunction with natural treatments and then taper off the medication as the nutritional supplements begin to aid your total condition. Naturally, these adjustments would have to occur with the approval and under the direction of your physician.

What To Do About Side Effects?

Stehlin (1990) suggests the following guidelines for lessening the side effects of NSAIDs:

- In general, all NSAIDs should be taken with food. It's often helpful to eat, take the pill, then eat again.
- In order to control the development of ulcers while you're taking NSAIDs, your doctor may prescribe Misoprostol. If you are pregnant, your doctor will suggest a different medication.
- Drink at least eight ounces of water when taking tablets or capsules to keep the lining of the esophagus and stomach from becoming irritated.

- Don't lie down for thirty minutes or so after taking your medicine. Gravity helps assure that the pill passes through the esophagus (food tube).
- Always take the exact dose prescribed by your doctor. Never double it, even if you miss a scheduled dose.
- Pregnant or breast-feeding women should not take NSAIDs unless specifically directed to and monitored by a doctor.
- Do not use alcohol while taking NSAIDs. Doing so increases the risk of stomach problems.
- Don't combine acetaminophen (such as Tylenol) with NSAIDs unless specifically directed to do so by your doctor.
- Inform your doctor of all other medications you are taking, whether prescription or over-the-counter, so it can be determined whether one drug will interact with another.
- If you are having surgery, inform your doctor or dentist that you are on NSAID therapy, even a low dose.
- Avoid driving or operating machinery when you are taking NSAIDs for they may cause drowsiness, confusion, or dizziness in a small number of patients.
- Be careful in direct sunlight. Your skin's sensitivity may be increased during NSAID therapy.

Suggestions for Taking Medications

Physicians make the very best decisions that they possibly can, but in many cases it is very, very difficult to prescribe the proper medication with the right dose to be taken at the right time for the right reasons. Very often physicians are unaware of some of the side effects of medications, or they may not be aware of the drug history of a patient, or they aren't told what drugs may have been prescribed alongside other drugs being suggested at any particular time. Also, many physicians are now required to prescribe a limited number of drugs, even if another one may be better suited for your needs.

These are all very good reasons for you to be well informed and educated about the medications that may be prescribed for you. Also be sure that your physician has a complete history of any drugs that you have used or are currently taking. The following are some guidelines and questions to ask as you work with your physician on the proper regimen for prescriptions (Theodosakis, 1990):

- Why do I need this drug?
- What are the possible side effects, from the most common to the very least?
- Who is most likely to suffer these side effects?
- What early signs will warn me that the side effects may be striking?
- Is there another medicine better suited to my needs?
- Is there a generic version of the drug that would work just as well for me but costs less?
- How many times a day should I take the medication? When? Should I take it with food or water, or on an empty stomach?
- Are there any foods or drinks I should avoid while taking this drug?
- Are there any activities I should restrict or avoid while taking this drug?
- How soon should the drug begin working?
- How will I know it's working?
- Assuming it works, how long should I continue taking it?
- If it doesn't work, how long before we try something else?
- Is there a nondrug treatment I might try?

Be certain that your physician is aware of your complete regimen, including your healthful diet, the nutritional supplements you're taking, and any other drugs that you are currently taking. If your physician prescribes medications for your condition, ask about supplemental nutrients.

CHAPTER 3

Curing Fibromyalgia: The 9-Step Action Plan

"Remember that your obstacles, crises and setbacks can become your greatest assets, if you so choose."

Dr. Joe M. Elrod

Magnesium, manganese, the powerful bioflavonoids and antioxidants, along with the phytonutrients described will do absolutely wonderful things for your fibromyalgia symptoms. However, they are only part of the fibromyalgia cure. The majority of fibromyalgia sufferers I have worked with had experienced a traumatic emotional experience, usually of a very long duration. Most of them were not exercising properly, were not following a very healthful diet, did not have very good stress coping skills, and typically did not ingest the proper vitamins, minerals and nutrients. As a result of these experiences and lifestyle, their immune system began to break down over time and they began to experience the fibromyalgia symptoms.

I have been most successful using the Nine-Step Action Plan to help dozens of fibromyalgia sufferers reverse their symptoms and begin almost immediately on a return trek to restoring their health and vitality. Just a word of warning: this series of steps is not a cure-all and it does not work 100 percent for everyone, but it is the most complete and effective regimen I can recommend for reversing fibromyalgia. Additionally, because of its all natural emphasis, the potential for harm and side effects is almost nonexistent. The steps do not necessarily have to occur in order—they will all be going on simultaneously.

1. Consultation with your physician or health professional
2. Returning to deep restful sleep
3. Detoxify and cleanse the body
4. Boost the immune system
5. Adopt a healthful nutrition program
6. Utilize nutritional supplementation
7. Adhere to a life-sustaining, healing exercise program
8. Develop and utilize good stress-coping skills
9. Employ the power of positive thinking

Action Step One

CONSULTATION WITH YOUR PHYSICIAN OR HEALTH PROFESSIONAL

Since there are many physical conditions that are very similar or coincide with fibromyalgia, the symptoms sometimes are very confusing to the patient and to the physician—beware of self-diagnosis. With fibromyalgia, or any other chronic condition, it is vitally important that one get a correct diagnosis and prescription for treatment. For example, I was recently conducting a seminar in Atlanta and was approached by a couple who inquired about fibromyalgia and its symptoms. I was informed that the husband was suffering with fibromyalgia. I talked with them for some time, asked many of the questions I normally ask, and then did some diagnosis by palpation to discover the gentleman had pain only on one area of the body. He did not have fibromyalgia but instead had a problem with his rotator cuff in the right shoulder. He needed to get help from an orthopedic specialist for proper diagnosis and treatment.

Following this example, if you suspect fibromyalgia, be certain to get a thorough evaluation and have a consultation with a medical doctor, preferably a rheumatologist who has experience with the condition. Finally, even if you are reasonably certain that you have fibromyalgia, be sure to consult with your physician and have an examination before starting this program.

Action Step Two

RETURNING TO DEEP RESTFUL SLEEP

Deep and restful sleep is one of the keys to restoring your health and returning to an active, vibrant lifestyle. Deep sleep (level 4) allows the body to replenish on a daily basis and helps defend against chronic fatigue, stress, depression, and the breaking down of the immune system which protects against the onset of illnesses such as fibromyalgia.

As a result of a lack of deep sleep and fatigue, most fibromyalgia patients feel totally drained of energy. The fatigue symptom can be mild in some and incapacitating in others. Ninety percent of the patients with fibromyalgia describe moderate to severe fatigue similar to the exhaustion experienced with the flu. Most frequently the fatigue is more of a problem than the pain. Most fibromyalgia sufferers will have difficulty sleeping, either awakening several times during the night or engaging in light sleep, and generally will wake up feeling very tired. In a research study done within a sleep lab, researchers found that fibromyalgia patients could fall asleep without much difficulty because of fatigue, however their deep sleep level was constantly interrupted by bursts of "awake-like" brain activity. Many fibromyalgia patients have an associated deep sleep disorder called the "alpha-EEG anomaly" (Hauri, 1973). They appear to spend the night in and out of light sleep, awakening in the early morning with an unrefreshed feeling. Most of them are unaware that their fatigue is a result of never entering the stage 4 sleep that is so necessary for health and vitality. Your potential for returning to deep, replenishing sleep is greatly enhanced if you will utilize the following suggestions:

- *Stick to your regular exercise program.* Remember that exercise is the most effective way to dissipate the energy produced by stress and is essential for reducing tension. Also remember that exercise will strengthen and restore the flexibility to your muscles, eventually reducing and eliminating the pain associated with fibromyalgia. Exercise also stimulates the production of T-cells to boost the immune system and releases healing, uplifting endorphins. All of these factors will assist with inducing deep sleep. Remember not to exercise too late in the day as this could disrupt your sleep.
- *Utilize your good stress coping skills.* Take mini-breaks during the day and practice your deep breathing and muscle relaxation exercises. Also take fifteen minutes periodically during the day to do some stretching exercises. These will increase blood flow, refresh and energize you.
- *Take time to play.* Make sure you have enough fun in your life. Go on a picnic with your family, take your dog for a walk, or go to a movie—whatever it is that you enjoy! Relaxation and good times are therapeutic and rewarding.

- *Cut down on caffeine and alcohol, especially late in the day and at night.* Having a nightcap before going to bed can actually leave you tired and listless the next morning.
- *Spend the last hour before going to bed winding down.* Take a relaxing hot bath, review your goals, focus on everything that's joyful, good, happy, and positive, and read from stimulating and motivating sources.
- *Adhere to your healthful nutrition and supplementation regimens.* Some simple healthful guidelines such as lowering fat, limiting fried foods, increasing fiber and modifying sugar intake will enhance better sleep. Eating more fruits and vegetables, along with taking a healthy regimen of vitamins and minerals, tends to have a cleansing and balancing effect that works to increase the potential for sleep.
- *Try the adaptogenic herb ginseng.* More than four thousand years ago the Chinese made claims that this herb tranquilized the spirit, calmed agitation of the mind, and warded off harmful influences while restoring and revitalizing the internal organs. Adaptogens, essential to plant and animal life, must adapt to changing temperatures, light patterns, and a variety of other stresses. Research studies in Europe and Japan have confirmed ginseng's ability to reduce stress and improve mental function. The most common forms of ginseng are Korean, Chinese, and Siberian. Each type works a little differently, so take as directed on the label. Choose a product with a high percentage of ginsenosides, the active ingredients (Tenney, 1995).
- *Develop a regular schedule.* For most people, it helps to develop a routine of retiring and rising at about the same times on a daily basis. It is typically devastating for the fibromyalgia sufferer to get out of a routine and retire later than normal and miss one good night's sleep. Some of the symptoms return almost immediately with such a disruption.
- *Try chamomile tea and melatonin.* A half hour before retir-

ing, drink one cup of chamomile tea and take 2-6 milligrams of melatonin. Melatonin is produced by the pineal gland which is embedded behind your eyes in the brain. As light fades away and darkness comes about, this small gland secretes melatonin which calms, relaxes and promotes sleep. (Experiment with different amounts until you find what's right for you.) Valerian and passionflower are also two relaxing and calming herbs that can be tried.

- *Sleep in a comfortable, quiet environment.* Wakefulness and sleeping are regulated by circadian rhythms in a twenty-four hour cycle. This cycle is regulated by exposure to light and the secretion of hormones, particularly melatonin. Utilize heavy curtains to block out light and use music or recorded nature sounds (e.g. waves or waterfalls) to block outside distracting noises.

Action Step Three

DETOXIFY AND CLEANSE THE BODY

The total cleansing process includes blood cleansing, digestive tract cleansing, colon cleansing, and total body cleansing. The key is to utilize healthful nutrition and natural nutrient supplementation to thoroughly cleanse the body, removing harmful toxins so that the immune system is boosted and fully functioning for its health restoring and maintenance process. The following are suggested supplements to aid you in your detoxification and cleansing program:

- *Red Clover:* This herb is a natural blood purifier and builder and is more potent in its liquid form. It has been used to give the body strength and energy and to protect and strengthen the immune system. Some of the better red clover products will have some supplemental herbs added such as echinacea, licorice root, cascara bark, and rosemary. It is recommended to take one teaspoon twice daily with a large glass of water or fruit juice. Remember, within your health and healing regimen you are to drink a minimum of eight to ten eight-ounce glasses of water daily.

- *Pau d' Arco:* This agent acts is a natural blood cleanser and builder. It has antibiotic properties which can aid in destroying bioinfections in the body. It helps combat cancer and has been used to strengthen the immune system.

- *Apple cider vinegar:* This is one of the best body purifiers and cleansers, especially when used in its organic form. It is usually a very potent formula and is best used when mixed with a healthy juice or purified water. (Recommended dosage is one tablespoon twice a day.)

- *Acidophilus:* This is a digestive tract and colon cleanser used to replace good bacteria in the digestive tract and to fight disease and infection. Cultured yogurt (with live cultures) is an excellent source of acidophilus.

- *Goldenseal:* Goldenseal assists in boosting a sluggish glandular system and promotes hormonal production. It is a very powerful nutrient that goes directly into the blood stream and assists in regulating liver function. Goldenseal is reported to act as a natural insulin by providing the body with nutrients necessary to produce its own insulin. This aids metabolism and energy production and makes goldenseal a most effective supplement for fibromyalgia. It also acts as a natural antibiotic to stop infections and kill poisons in the body.

- *Magnesium and Malic acid:* Make certain that you use a combination of magnesium and malic acid in your healing regimen. This combination is the key to restoring the efficiency of the energy production process that physiologically stimulates the healing process. Malic acid is a food supplement found in citrus fruits and is very plentiful in apples. Some studies have found that it assists energy, metabolism, muscle health, and is most helpful in fibromyalgia. Take as recommended.

Action Step Four

BOOST THE IMMUNE SYSTEM

This component is part of the healing regimen because additional boosting of the immune system is always helpful and might be essential. Remember that a weakened immune system is the primary problem with systemic conditions such as fibromyalgia. Of course, a healthful nutrition program, an exercise program, some stress coping techniques, and healthful supplementation will all boost the immune system tremendously. The following are some very powerful immune boosters that will assist with your return to health and vitality:

- *Pycnogenol (proanthocyanadins):* This is a very powerful antioxidant extracted from grape seed and maritime bark. According to researchers, grape seed extract appears to be a potent immune booster and is fifty times stronger than vitamin E. Pycnogenol strengthens collagen (the reinforcement bars of the cells), improves circulation, and enhances the permeability of cell walls. It enhances metabolism and promotes a healing effect in the body. Suggested dosage is 50-200 milligrams daily, depending upon the severity of the condition.
- *Bee pollen:* Bee pollen is very high in protein and is considered one of the most complete foods that we can consume. It contains rich sources of vitamins, minerals, amino acids, proteins, enzymes, and fats. Bee pollen aids hormone

imbalances and is very useful to the fibromyalgia patient because it helps to improve the appetite, normalize intestinal activity, strengthen capillary walls, and offset the effects of drugs and pollutants, Bee pollen is also effective for healing colitis and improving anemia. A very high grade of bee pollen, preferably in granular form, should be sought out and can generally be found in health food stores. A precautionary statement for those with allergies is that you may need to start with as little as one granule per day in order to build up a tolerance to any allergic reaction. Suggested dosage is one teaspoon of granules per day following buildup.

- *Coenzyme Q-10:* This is a powerful antioxidant and food supplement that increases circulation and is used by the muscles for energy and to enhance metabolism. Co Q-10 is believed to be about twenty times stronger than vitamin E. Suggested dosage is 50 mg minimum per day.

- *Echinacea:* Echinacea is another powerful nutrient that stimulates the immune response and helps the body increase its ability to resist infection, produce white blood cells, and purify the blood. Echinacea is considered to be a natural antibiotic.

- *Selenium and Zinc:* These two trace minerals are very powerful antioxidants and are essential to boosting the immune system and the healing process. Selenium works synergistically with other nutrients, especially vitamin E. It assists the body in utilizing oxygen and helps with normal growth function and healing. Two good sources of selenium are alfalfa and kelp. Zinc helps with the absorption of vitamins in the body and assists in the formation of skin, hair, and nails. It is an essential part of many enzymes involved in digestion, metabolism and the creation of energy. Zinc is also essential to the growth process. Vitamin A must be present for zinc to be properly absorbed by the body. Ginseng and kelp are good sources of zinc. Recommended dosage for selenium is 250 micrograms per day and for zinc 30 milligrams per day.

Action Step Five

ADOPT A HEALTHFUL NUTRITION PROGRAM

Nutrition is a critical factor in the treatment and healing of fibromyalgia. Some nutritional guidelines will enhance your chances of recovering from fibromyalgia as well as protecting you against cancer, heart disease, arthritis, diabetes, and stroke. For the most efficient health recovery and healing regimen and for the body to function at peak performance you need an excellent balance and a wide variety of foods that include complex carbohydrates, the helpful fats, protein, fiber, vitamins, minerals, phytochemicals, and the potent bioflavonoids.

Remember the most healthful eating patterns are eating five or six times daily; boiling, broiling, baking and steaming while limiting fried foods; and never skipping meals, especially breakfast. Choose foods that provide the necessary increased fiber and fluid, the higher quality fats, the complex carbohydrates, necessary proteins and the vitamins and minerals necessary for optimal health and for combating the fibromyalgia symptoms. Chapter 5 provides a complete nutritional and supplemental program for your health and recovery.

(Note: Look for the power foods list at the end of the nutrition chapter selecting those with vitamins, minerals, bioflavonoids, and phytonutrients that are needed for the most effective health and healing program. Finally, refer to the nutrition chapter for the 21-day detoxification program and the healthful daily regimen you should follow.)

Action Step Six

UTILIZE NUTRITIONAL SUPPLEMENTATION

Do you need nutritional supplements? Authorities now agree that the average American diet no longer provides the needed nutrition for a foundation of good health. Half of all foods eaten in America are over processed and convenience foods have little if any nutritional value. Eighty percent of middle class American children and 90 percent of American adults are severely malnourished. Both children and adults choose to eat for taste, cost, and convenience. Coffee, white bread, and sugar are the most popular and most often consumed foods. Ironically, most of our pets eat a far better, more nutritionally rich daily diet of proteins, carbohydrates, appropriate fats, vitamins, and minerals than do most American children or adults (Carper, 1995).

Good nutrition provides the antioxidants, bioflavonoids, and phytonutrients needed for health and vitality. Antioxidants are known for their special role as a preventative aid in controlling excess oxidation and free radical damage. Free radicals are unstable molecules produced from oxygen and fats. Antioxidants are necessary nutrients and enzymes that buffer or break down free radicals to prevent them from damaging healthy cells (Tenney, 1995). Research has pointed out that polyunsaturated fats are thought to be easily converted into free radicals. Oily salad dressings, fried foods, and junk foods contain high amounts of polyunsaturated. Most researchers believe that the aging process, some forms of heart disease, cancer, diabetes, and yes, even fibromyalgia are related to free radical damage in the cells.

Highly refined and processed foods contain pollutants and chemical toxins. Fruits and vegetables, unless grown organically, will receive pesticide treatment and be exposed to even more toxins. The water we use, as well as the air we breathe, contains pollutants. Meats are often treated with antibiotics and hormones. These are all reasons why we need nutritional supplementation. Nutrients boost the antioxidant defense system and help protect the body from these environmental pollutants and toxins. (See Chapters 5 and 8 for more information.)

Action Step Seven

ADHERE TO A LIFE-SUSTAINING, HEALING EXERCISE PROGRAM

Exercise is one of the key components in the health and healing regimen for those with existing fibromyalgia. Exercise improves muscle tone as it increases a nourishing flow of blood into the tissues. It increases flexibility and/or the range of motion, increases the healing endorphins in the immune system, and enhances the production of T-cells that are highly effective in the efficient autoimmune system. Exercise also stimulates serotonin and the growth hormone. The right exercises are essential to weight control as well as to the reduction of pain and the increase of mobility of the fibromyalgia patient. Another outstanding benefit of exercise to the fibromyalgia patient is the improved health of the supportive structures and joints. At one time it was thought that exercise actually caused arthritis; however, we now know regular exercise is an excellent means of helping to keep joints healthy. (See Chapter 6.)

Action Step Eight

DEVELOP AND UTILIZE GOOD
STRESS-COPING SKILLS

Effective stress coping techniques can assist the fibromyalgia patient in fighting stress and depression. It is very important to understand the difference between stress and depression so that effective stress coping techniques can be employed. Stress is the response of the mind, body, and emotions to everyday happenings and the pressures of life. It is also important to recognize that stress is not the actual event, but rather our interpretation of and emotional reaction to the event. For example, a very active person might find a stress fracture injury very traumatic while the next person may find it an opportunity to rest up and refresh the body while recovering. The situations are similar, but it's how the individuals respond to the situation that determines the stress impact (O'Koon, 1996). The list below contains some guidelines for a healthful stress coping program:

- Boost your nutrition by eating more frequently, four to five times a day, and choosing an abundance of complex carbohydrates and high fiber foods such as whole grains, whole grain breads and cereals, rice, pasta, beans, peas, and potatoes, along with plenty of fresh fruits and vegetables. Only 20 percent of your total food volume should be fat. Avoid sugar, caffeine, and stay away from sugar-laden foods.
- Vitamin and mineral supplements of any antioxidant combination will boost the immune system and enhance the cellular cleansing process by maintaining and invigorating cellular energy, cardiovascular awareness, and youthful vitality.

49

- Get regular exercise. Exercise aerobically by cycling, walking or swimming a minimum of four to five times per week. Include stretching and muscle toning exercises two to three days per week. Joint stretching and muscle toning exercises will be very beneficial, and remember that exercising regularly will increase the potential for the fibromyalgia victim to move into deep sleep while resting.

- Balance rest and relaxation with your exercise and activity. Be sure to get adequate amounts of sleep, focus on the positive, work at sleeping peacefully by going through your relaxation exercises while visualizing your goals. Remember that rest and relaxation will help to reduce muscle tension which will help in reducing pain. It is also important to avoid prescription tranquilizers and sleeping medications of the benzodiazeprene group. While these may help you get to sleep, they will suppress deep sleep and often make fibromyalgia symptoms worse the next day. Alcohol or narcotic pain medications taken in the evenings have the same effect on deep sleep and should also be avoided.

- Practice good stress management techniques. Don't over extend yourself, always plan ahead for difficult tasks, and remember to ask for help whenever needed. Limit your responsibilities and activities to easily manageable levels.

- Be especially moderate with caffeine and alcoholic beverages. Do not use drugs unless necessitated and prescribed by your doctor.

- Ingest a reasonable number of calories to enhance your weight loss and/or weight maintenance program.

Action Step Nine

EMPLOY THE POWER OF POSITIVE THINKING

Positive thinking can do more for an ill person than many medications. There are many people who have experienced drastic change in their physical condition simply by choosing to perceive things differently; in essence, you change your attitude, your expectations and your vision of yourself and your condition.

CASE HISTORY

The following is an example of one of my former patients who was able to effectively overcome her fibromyalgia by following this nine-step plan.

Janice, a 38-year-old married mother of three, worked very hard at her job teaching seventh grade. She was always on the go but felt happy and seemed healthy. Even with work and home responsibilites, she still managed to attend aerobics classes three days a week. Then, almost suddenly, one morning when she attempted to get out of bed, she experienced a dull, aching pain in her neck and shoulder region for seemingly no reason whatsoever. At first, the pain only struck in the early morning as she was getting up, but very soon it began to hurt during the day—while standing and teaching in the classroom, while sitting at her desk, and finally even while she was sleeping. There seemed to be no real pattern to the pain, except that it steadily grew worse and seemed to spread to other parts of her body.

Fortunately, Janice had excellent medical insurance and made an appointment to see her physician. After an exhaustive testing session absolutely nothing showed up. Her blood work seemed to be normal, her blood pressure was okay, nothing positive resulted on any test for specific parts of the body, so she was told by her physician that apparently there was nothing wrong. She was eventually advised to just take Tylenol. But the pain continued to spread to other parts of her body and she had more and more difficulty sleeping so she was taken off Tylenol and put on ibuprofen. Her physician eventually told her that it seemed there was not much that could be done. Her family didn't really understand the problem either since the medical tests had not resulted in anything. It was sort of a catch-22 where a very painful and frustrating situation seemed to have her caught between her family, her physician, and her job.

Less than two years after the pain and stiffness first appeared in the morning, Janice was forced to stop doing many of the things she had previously done for her three small children. Nor did she have the energy or stamina to do as much with the house or for her husband. She was also beginning to be very limited as to what she could do with her job because of fatigue and anxiety as a result of a lack of proper rest.

After moving from stress and anxiety into depression, Janice had all but given up hope as to what to do about the pain or getting better. Then she heard about some natural nutrients that might be of some benefit to her. She began to take 800 I.U. of vitamin E, 1000 mg of vitamin C, and 25,000 I.U. of beta-carotene on a daily basis, along with 50 mg of coenzyme Q-10 and a combination of magnesium and malic acid. On the advice of a nutritionist, she changed her eating patterns drastically and began to walk fifteen to twenty minutes per day. Over a period of four to six weeks she progressed to the point where she was walking from forty-five minutes to one hour each day. After about six weeks on the program she began to realize that she was sleeping better, the pain was beginning to subside, and she was gradually moving back toward her normal activities. After about six months on this program, Janice was about 90 percent back to normal, excited about life, and making continuous progress toward returning to her health and vitality.

I am happy to report that dozens upon dozens of people that I have put on the four-pronged program presented in this book have made progress similar to Janice's. Also, physicians across the United States and around the world are beginning to learn and understand more about nutrients and supplements, nutrition programs, life-sustaining exercise programs, and good stress coping programs. Little by little they are beginning to prescribe them for their patients with the same excellent results.

Chapter 4

The Mind-Body Connection

"Each patient carries his own doctor inside him."
Albert Schweitzer

"I have learned never to underestimate the capacity of the human mind and body to regenerate—even when prospects seem most wretched. The life force may be the least understood force on this earth."
Dr. Norman Cousins

In the second century the Greek physician Galan noted that disease is a consequence of psychic imbalance. For more than a millennium that belief prevailed in the practice of medicine, until modern medical science rejected the idea that mental and emotional states influence the body's disease-fighting capacity. However, about 25 years ago, the connection between physiological factors and immune functions was revived and seriously examined. In fact, the belief that this connection exists has birthed the field of investigation called *psychoneuroimmunology* (PNI). PNI scholars and researchers focus primarily on how the brain and the body's immune system communicate.

The hypothalamus (the brain's autonomic center) and the pituitary gland (the body's master gland) are connected by a rich network of blood vessels. The discovery of this network has helped researchers understand how thoughts and emotions affect the immune system. The fact that the hormones of stress directly influence the immune response has been suspected for years by immunologists. Several research studies in recent years have indicated positive links between immune response and emotional factors. Research has also borne out that people being described as helpless, sad, unassertive, hopeless, passive, and fearful have shown greater incidences of cancer.

There is much evidence to indicate that communication exists between the brain and the immune system. The lymph nodes are one of the immune systems principal groups of organs. They are filled with nerve fibers that act like telephone trunk lines; for instance, the lymph nodes send and receive messages to and from the entire body. Special chemicals called "neurotransmitters" attach themselves to immune cells and influence their disease-fighting potential.

Psychoneuroimmunology researcher, Dr. Candace Pert, contends that brain cells produce small protein-like chemicals called neuropeptides to provide the chemical basis of emotion. Neuropeptides have powerful mood stimulating effects, and high concentrations of them are found in the limbic system of the brain, thought to be the "control center" of emotions. Endorphines, which are 200 times more powerful than morphine, are examples of neuropeptides. Intense and persistent periods of negative emotions such as fear, depression, grieving, and helplessness have been shown to suppress normal immune functions. On the other hand, research has shown that we can strengthen the immune system with confidence, happiness, and laughter as positive emotions. To achieve the highest level of health that we are capable of reaching, we absolutely need to establish a positive thought structure as our normal daily attitude. This program is designed to assist you in achieving just that.

It is a very interesting question indeed: why would mother nature link negative stress with the immune system? There are several possible explanations that have been offered by immunologists, but the most widely accepted one points to the preservation of energy. Temporarily diverting energy away from the internal immune struggles constantly waging throughout the body commits more energy to be summoned and garnered to face the perceived threat from outside. The greater the "perceived" threat and the negative emotion, the greater the degree of immune suppression.

Psychological Stress		Psychological Intervention (creating changed perceptions of ourselves and our problems)	
Depression, Despair		Hope, Anticipation	
Limbic System		Limbic System	
Hypothalamic Activity	Pituitary Activity	Hypothalamic Activity	Pituitary Activity
Immune System (anti-cancer mechanisms)	Endocrine System (hormonal imbalance)	Immune System	Endocrine System (restores hormonal balance)
Suppression of immune activity	Increase in abnormal cells	Increase in immune activity	Decrease in abnormal cells
Cancer Growth		Cancer Regression	

Table 2: *Perception of an Event* (Simonton, O. et al, 1992)

Very often when we are feeling sick or weak, I believe that it is nature's way of getting our attention. It truly is as though we have an internal "psychiatrist" who is trying to get our attention to help us make better decisions. *I truly believe that the condition of fibromyalgia is more directly related to stress*

57

and trauma as causative factors than any other one thing. If we would really stop and think about it, the mind has a much, much greater influence that we realize. I know for certain that I can remember times when I was under a great deal of stress, I would eventually catch a cold, and I can also remember times that I have made a commitment that I needed to keep, I would simply not allow myself to become sick because I could not "afford" to. I also remember times when I was exposed to a virus or other illnesses that were running rampant and I would not contract these because of a mental determination, along with a stronger immune system.

The ability to have control over our wellness and the ability to choose to be healthy and fully functioning is a new science growing in popularity. Scientists all over the world such as psychiatrists, endocrinologists, neuroscientists, immunologists, and microbiologists have united their fields of expertise and created a new field called psychoneuroimmunology. A straight-forward description of this field would state that this is a field that is concerned with the mind and how it can affect our immune system's complex network of vessels, internal organs, and white blood cells. One of the really fascinating facts in this area indicates that the vital body systems, the brain and the immune system, communicate with and influence one another. For instance, if your brain allows a stress level to get out of control, this can have a seriously detrimental impact on the immune system, which in turn can suppress its ability to fight disease. Another way to express this is to say if you are chronically distressed, anxious, or up-tight, then these very emotions can manifest themselves over the long term as heart disease, cancer, arthritis, and yes, even fibromyalgia. It is extremely interesting to note that on the other hand, well-managed stress can help keep your immune system healthy; if we are well-adjusted, happy, and content, the body will maintain its disease fighting forces at peak capacity.

It seems apparent that we can prevent the onset of disease or lessen the impact of a disease or stimulate the healing of a condition of a disease by adjusting our mental outlook. Russian scientists were the first to express this viewpoint. Although they were sternly ridiculed in the beginning by some of the conservative immunologists in the field who argued that immune responses should be observed in the test tube with no intervention from the mind whatsoever. However, in the past ten years a neurophysiologist at the National Institute of Health in Bethesda, Maryland, Dr. Novera Herbert Spector, states that new research makes it very clear that attitudes can matter and make a significant difference. My personal research and results with clients supports totally Dr. Spector's hypothesis.

A husband/wife radio therapist/psychiatrist team, Dr. O. Carl Simonton and Stephanie Simonton, have developed a whole person approach to combat disease. The Simonton Method calls for the patient to alter emotions, expectations, and attitudes in combating disease. Daily exercises for relaxation, imaging, and physical activity are very important to this process, according to the Simontons. The Simontons verify in their research that an individual's wellness or illness involves not simply the physiology of the body, but rather the whole person which incorporates both the body and the mind. The basic premise behind this theory is that *mental therapy uses emotions to prod certain brain chemicals into stimulating the body's defense systems against the invading disease.* This situation of endorphins and catacholomines and the T-cells from the thymus gland enhance the immune system's ability to fight disease and assist an individual in getting well. I suggest some relaxation, imaging, and positive thinking exercises at the end of this section.

Dr. Carol Ann Sperling, a clinical psychologist and director of the Cancer Counseling Institute in Bethesda, Maryland, states that if one gets angry and that particular emotion does not get discharged, and if the resulting hormonal products and small particles such as neurotransmitters and endorphines do not get used, then this in turn cannot benefit the immune system. Dr. Sperling goes further to say that these chemicals sink down, yet they don't go away and the residue can become toxic in our bodies.

Dr. Norman Cousins

In his book, *The Anatomy of An Illness,* Dr. Norman Cousins describes how he made a miraculous recovery from a long debilitating illness. Laughter was one of the tools that Cousins used in a conscious effort to mobilize and to enhance his will to live. Dr. Cousins who was a senior lecturer in medicine at UCLA and a long-time editor of *Saturday Review,* had a disease called ankylosing spondylitis. Dr. Cousins was told by a specialist that he had a one in 500 chance of recovering from this progressive and incurable disease. Dr. Cousins agreed with the specialist on one condition: that if he lingered in a hospital, harassed with taking pain medications and going through x-rays, that indeed certainly would be the case. He therefore checked out of the hospital and proceeded to work with his doctor to devise his own treatment plan. His plan consisted of three parts:

1. He stopped all medications believing that pain killers have the potential to inhibit the body's self-healing processes.
2. He took mega doses of vitamin C intravenously.
3. Perhaps the most important part, according to some of the research that we are citing here, he set out to arrest the disease process by cultivating the positive emotions of laughter, faith, love, hope, and the will to live.

He noted that ten minutes of genuine, deep laughter would give him at least two hours of deep restful pain-free sleep. His healing method was most unconventional, but miraculously proved to be most successful and now the once dying Dr. Norman Cousins has restored health and plays his two favorite sports of golf and tennis regularly.

THE SUCCESS ATTITUDE

Attitude is generally described as our feelings or perception about circumstances, other people, and more importantly, about ourselves. Attitude is the one factor that causes more people not to achieve and get to where they want to be with health, family, finances, and career than any other factor.

It is critical for us to understand how our attitude can make us or break us. Our attitude influences our smile, our handshake, our appearance, the words we speak, as well as the actions we take or don't take. It is all these things put together that determine whether we will be successful, and just how successful we will become, whether we will get well and stay well.

So then, this process outlined for you in this section can be vital for your recovering and healing. Let me ask you what your thoughts might be about being healthy, being restored completely, and also what are your thoughts on a consistent basis? Are you thinking only healthy, recovering, alive thoughts or do you focus on the negative as you proceed through each da?. Remember, you have a choice. Do you expect to get sicker or are your expectations to get well? Are you visualizing health and vitality, happiness, and a pain-free body? Remember that your body will respond chemically and manifest your thoughts. If you think healthy, positive thoughts, you will begin to create a momentum toward health and vitality. It is true, you can literally choose to be healthy, happy, and successful.

At this time, you may wish to consider that famous John Dorphine quotation: "The mind is its own place, and in itself can make heaven of hell, or a hell of heaven." I have decided to include this section in the book because I have an unshakable belief in the power of will, faith, and hope in assisting with all types of problems, whether they be mental or physical, or a combination of the two. For more than 15 years now, I have done counseling on an individual basis, as well as on a group basis, and many of my clients have benefited greatly from the outlined procedures here.

The following four major components are the ingredients for building the positive success attitude. When you effectively put the following together, then you can and will possess the attitude and prowess to get well, be successful financially or accomplish whatever you choose to do:

- Desire and Belief
- Positive Self-Expectancy
- Visualization and Concentration
- Preparation for Winning

Desire and Belief

I have chosen to place desire and belief together for an important purpose. These, in my opinion, are the two central ingredients to motivation and achievement. All achievement and success that is meaningful has its beginning with desire and is brought to fruition only if one believes strongly enough (i.e. Dr. Cousins) that it will happen.

The most important realization about desire is that it must come from within. You cannot and will not get well or become successful simply because your parents, your spouse, your coach, your supervisor, or manager want you to, or because someone else has recognized your incredible ability. Every answer to every problem or the key to any solution is within you and your will and desire to succeed must come from within. The more desire you have, the less you limit your potential and the more you will be able to accomplish. This chapter is included spefically to help you realize your potential for *getting well*, being happy and becoming successful.

The second key ingredient for this section is belief. Belief or faith is an attribute that all positive people exhibit. Nothing of any great significance was ever accomplished without the component of belief. The basis for belief is confidence and positive thinking. Positive, successful people exude an air of confidence and appear to be in complete control most of the time. It is the quality of belief that brings about a confidence that enables one to perform well, even under pressure. In fact, it is usually those without a strong sense of belief and those who lack confidence who generally fall apart under pressure.

Roger Staubach was asked how the Dallas Cowboys always seemed to be successful in coming from behind and winning game after game in the last two minutes. Roger responded, "At the end of every practice, we run a two-minute drill and our goal is to run 60 perfect pass plays. If someone jumps count or drops the ball on the 52nd pass play, for instance, we start back at number one until we run 60 perfect plays. Then in the game, you see, it is second nature for us to run the two-minute drill to perfection. We have instilled such an air of confidence and belief, it's really hard not to accomplish what we set out to do."

Positive Self-Expectancy

It has been said that one of the most outward, recognizable characteristics of healthy, successful people is positive self-expectancy. Research done on the subconscious mind and human performance in the past century has literally revolutionized our thinking on the power of the mind and human capability. In fact, this research stimulated William James, the renowned psychologist, to state the following: "The greatest discovery of my lifetime has been that, man can alter his life by altering his attitude."

Dr. Joseph Murphy in his wonderful book, The Power of *Your Subconscious Mind,* explains in intricate detail the psychological power of expectancy. For instance, he explains the passing-over technique which consists essentially of inducing the subconscious mind to take over your request of what you want to happen as given it by the conscious mind. Dr. Murphy explains that this passing-over is best accomplished in the reverie-like state. In other words, this technique works especially well in a very quiet, relaxed state. This way, the kinetic energy of the subconscious produces positive, successful, pleasant thoughts. Dr. Murphy says, "Just know that in your deeper mind is Infinite Intelligence and Infinite Power, so calmly structure in your mind what you want to happen and vividly imagine it coming into fruition from that moment on."

Bruce Jenner, after having lost every event in the decathlon in Munich, was interviewed in the streets of the Olympic Village. He was asked what he would do now that his Olympic career was over. He replied, "I don't think you understand, I will win the decathlon in Montreal four years from now." With that image of positive self-expectation etched into his subconscious mind, Bruce set out, arising early every day and working persistently toward his goal of becoming the best athlete in the world, and won the decathlon in Montreal.

The power of positive self-expectation has been realized and recognized by mankind throughout the ages. Wise King Solomon in the 8th century B.C. stated, "As a man thinketh in his heart, so is he." Centuries later, Marcus Aurelius, the Roman emperor and philosopher, wrote "A man's life is what his thoughts make of it." In his research, Dr. Denis Waitley has reinforced that, "we will tend to perform the way we see ourselves in our mind's eye." Finally, Earl Nightingale, after a lifetime of research and study of human nature, was prompted to quote Emerson and conclude, "You will become what you think about all day long."

The power of expectation is both intrinsic and extrinsic. We not only respond and move toward our own expectations but, at the same time, we are impacted by the expectations of others for us. Our parents, spouses, teachers, supervisors, coaches, and peers have a marked influence on our efforts and accomplishments. So then, isn't it quite exciting to contemplate the fact that each of us has within us the built-in mechanism to utilize the above technique, through commitment; to get well, be happy, become successful?

Visualization and Concentration

Visualization is nothing more than mental imaging. All successful people have mastered the art of mental imaging and practice some form of visualization on a consistent basis. You can literally control your destiny by etching the images of the things you want to bring about on the subconscious mind. The mind is an amazing mechanism that functions like a heat-seeking missile. The images that we hold consistently in the mind, we will move toward and bring into reality. We can become only what we act as if and believe that we already are.

An example of this phenomenon working in an amazing way involves the story of a United States Air Force officer from Oregon who was captured and spent seven years in a Vietnamese prisoner-of-war camp. Before his capture he had been a par golfer. Approximately six weeks after his release, he was invited to play in the New Orleans Professional/Amateur Tournament and shot a 76, only four strokes over par. A reporter interviewed him and remarked that his feat was quite phenomenal since he had not touched a golf club in seven years. He explained that it was not a phenomenal feat at all, because he had played eighteen holes of golf in his mind every day for seven years. He explained that he visualized the course precisely, saw every fairway, bunker, and green vividly in his mind. He said that he studied every shot, selected every club very carefully and would imagine each swing whether it was a drive, chip, or putt with perfect technique.

Develop the habit of visualizing at various times: when sitting at your desk, before a meeting, during exercise, or while listening to motivational tapes. While showering and dressing in the morning are other suggested times to practice visualization. Picture yourself consistently as a healthy, vibrant individual enjoying the things related to your purpose, choice, and passion. Remember, that visualization and concentration develop confidence and help remove doubt and fear. This feeling of confidence combined with the visualization process enhances your positive attitude and promotes success and wellness.

PREPARING FOR RECOVERY

It is a foregone conclusion, successful people are made and not born. The reason people are successful is definitely not education or talent alone. There are thousands of educated derelicts, as well as thousands of people with great raw talent who have never accomplished anything above the average or mediocre.

The first thing to accept and understand then, is that you reach your goals and desired destinations through commitment, persistence, belief, and hard work. The leaders in sales spend hours daily on self-improvement, planning, and organizational skills. Colonel Sanders was told "no" 1009 times before receiving a "yes" on his chicken recipe that eventually led to his amazing success story. "Pistol Pete" Maravich was an All-American basketball player at LSU, averaging an amazing 44.8 points per game for his collegiate career. His scoring average still stands as an NCAA record after more than twenty years. Every day Pete would arrive at practice an hour or two before the regular practice time to work on his conditioning, shooting skills, and ball handling skills. He became the best through practice, practice, practice; not simply by being born talented. In all successful people you will discover a positive attitude. And within the positive attitude you will always find the ingredients of desire and belief, positive self-expectancy, the ability to visualize and concentrate, and a willingness to persevere as they prepare and expect to move toward their desired goal. Remember, you will become what you visualize and think about most often.

POSITIVE BEGINNINGS

One of the keys for success is to develop the positive habit pattern of awakening each day with a thankful heart and a positive, optimistic attitude with which to program the subconscious mind for total success throughout the day. Remember, as you first begin to gain consciousness in the early morning, the brain is functioning at the sub-conscious or alpha level and there are only 10-12 brain wave lengths per second. Therefore, whatever you program at this point or allow to be etched on the subconscious will go with you throughout the day. This is the point daily at which you decide whether you will be well, happy, optimistic, productive, successful, etc. Take the following prescription for a positive, uplifting, joyous, rewarding, productive day, every day!

EARLY MORNING

Awaken Early/Thankful Heart
Visualize Yourself a Winner
Inspirational Reading
Review Your Goals
Brainstorming/Idea Session
Brief Walk/Exercise
Shower/Mind Readiness
Heart Healthy Breakfast

COURSE OF THE DAY

Positive, Wholesome Thoughts
Pleasant Greeting and Smile to Everyone
Answer Greetings with "Wonderful," "Fantastic"
Offer Sincere Appreciation
Listen More, Talk Less
Work Your Plan/Schedule

Be Flexible
Exercise, Play and Relaxation
See Your Work as Pleasure
Moderate Lunch (50%)
Reasonable, Balanced Dinner
Family Time

LATE EVENING

Success Journal
Thankful Heart/Review Goals
Today's Success/Tomorrow's Plan
Inspirational Reading and/or Tape
Plan and Program for Tomorrow
Brainstorms/Ideas/Solutions

KEYS FOR SUCCESS

A lifetime of experience coupled with twenty-five years of research have yielded the answer to a question that intrigued me for the better part of my life: "Why do some achieve in such an extraordinary fashion, others fail so miserably, and the masses settle for the average or mediocre?" I discovered that many scholars and researchers have sought to answer the same question. We have all come to the same basic conclusion: there are common denominators that bring about extraordinary human achievement. The common denominators yielded by my experiences and research are listed below as the "Keys For Success." Each of the keys or concepts will be explained briefly on the subsequent pages. If you will embrace these principles and concepts and apply them, your chances for achieving health and success in all other areas will be enhanced tremendously.

Keys for Success

A. Establish Your Values
B. Get in Touch with Your Life's Purpose
C. Mold a Mission
D. Set and Write Your Goals
E. Establish and Write Your Action Plan
F. Visualize Yourself a Winner
G. Learn the Art of Motivation
H. Learn the Art of Communication
I. Employ the Power of a Thankful Heart
J. Become a Serious Student/Tap the Treasury of Ideas
K. Discover the Magic of Giving

Establish Your Values

One must identify and understand what is most important to them, what they value the most, and what they would fight for and defend. Until one establishes this baseline, it is impossible to set meaningful goals and choose direction in life.

Get in Touch with Your Life Purpose

Every individual possesses specific and unique gifts and talents to carry out a particular purpose in this life. In other words, every life has a purpose and will achieve total peace and contentment only if they are working and serving within their particular purpose. Engage your family members, friends, work associates, teammates, etc., to assist you in affirming your gifts and talents. This one thing will assist you more than any other in determining your life purpose. This and other techniques will be presented later to assist you in your purpose decisions in life (i.e., going on vacation, the promotion to vice-president, which civic club to join, going out for the team, taking a computer course, choosing your college major, your life vocation, or the person to marry).

Mold a Mission

Once your values are established and you have a feel for the talents and abilities that clue you to your life purpose, you can then begin to zero in on life and mold a mission. It does not occur to many people that they were given special gifts and traits with which they can excel. You were given the wherewithal to carve out your niche in life, so follow these steps and go for it. Many never realize it and never accomplish it because of never receiving the knowledge and facts being presented to you now. Most go to classes in school systems throughout the world from twelve to twenty years and never have a course that teaches the concepts in this chapter. Once you realize your life has a purpose and once you begin to move toward something you really desire, life gets exciting and you can begin to mold a mission (set life goals) that will get you up each morning with enthusiasm, which will ultimately stimulate the production of life-sustaining and healing hormones internally.

Set and Write Your Goals

One major mistake that many people make is that they attempt to set goals as the first step in the success procedure. We must first establish our values, begin to understand our purpose for existing and begin to mold a mission in life before we can adequately set and write our goals. It is then that writing goals carries a magic that etches them indelibly into our subconscious mind. Research has proven this important concept time and again: the images we hold constantly in our mind will eventually come to pass.

Ralph Waldo Emerson was referring to the immeasurable human potential when he wrote, "What lies before us and what lies behind us pales in significance when we realize what lies within us." The goal setting principles in this chapter are shared to assist you to realize the vast potential within. Once we begin to set goals, visions begin to be etched on the subconscious mind. As these visions become crystallized in our mind's eye, we begin to get excited about life and generate an enthusiasm that eventually results in action that transforms our dreams into reality. As we move toward accomplishment and begin to feel the exhilaration of the fulfillment of all that we were intended to be, we begin to experience the abundance and inner peace that has been promised in life.

GUIDELINES FOR GOAL SETTING

Principle One: Things won't change until you change. Make the commitment now to develop unusual habits. Consistent, productive, positive habits will lead to goal achievement and success. Successful people are not those without problems, they are simply those with persistent habits that they have learned and who are willing to solve their problems.

Principle Two: The goal setting process is tedious and time consuming. Make the commitment now to invest ample time for planning and structuring your life for success. Commit to developing unusual habits to support your time investment (i.e., reviewing and revising your goals frequently, arising early, being prompt, returning calls, completing assignments, always doing more than you're paid to do, develop a thankful attitude rather than a critical one, giving your time, money, and effort).

Principle Three: You won't get much by demand; it's what you do by performance that will yield results. It comes from within you, you have all the answers, gifts, talents within you to achieve your goals and your desires—get more out of you.

Principle Four: Don't wish it were easier, wish you were better. Remember that your obstacles, crises, and setbacks are your greatest assets. It is through overcoming these that you become stronger, wiser, better. Emerson said it so poetically when he stated, "When man sits on the cushions of comfort he goes to sleep, but when he sits on the needles of adversity he rises up to do great things."

Principle Five: It is not what happens to you (circumstances), it's how you respond to what happens that makes the difference in success and failure. Your experiences plus your responses have determined where you are, who you are, and what you are. E (experience) + R (response) = YOU.

Principle Six: Life is not a destination, it's a journey. The key to fulfillment in life is to realize that it's not what you get at the end that's important, but what you become in the process. Cervantes summed it up with great wisdom when he stated, "The road is much better than the end."

Establish and Write Your Action Plan

It has been written that the best plan in the world will not work if you won't. Without a plan of action, a goal remains in the dream category and will eventually fade away. *Remember that motivation and good positive feelings come after taking action.* Many are deceived into thinking that one gets motivated, then acts. This principle is illustrated by the fellow sitting before the wood stove and saying, "Give me some heat and I will then put some wood in you." As a further illustration, when you chop your own wood, you warm yourself twice. Finally, your action plan will be your daily road map. Could you imagine building a house without the plan? A builder would need to know the specifics of how many square feet, the exact materials, the style of home with every detail, in order to produce the desired home. This very book can serve as an action plan for your return to health and vitality, study it and make a commitment to follow the life restoring regimen.

Visualize Yourself a Winner

The most powerful mechanism we have available for success is the ability of the subconscious mind to imagine or visualize what we want to happen. Unfortunately, it works in the negative as well; we can literally destroy ourselves with worry, doubt and fear. Therefore, it is vital to train the subconscious to cancel out the negative and consistently harbor the positive.

Earlier in this chapter you were introduced to the Awaken and Program Success early-morning activity that will train you to develop the positive mental habit patterns characteristic of highly successful people. Psychology has proven that approximately twenty-one days are required to develop a habit. So, as you consistently visualize yourself a success, you will begin to walk, talk, and perform successfully in all areas of your life. As you learn to focus on your goals and the person you are becoming, your subconscious mind will attract, like a magnet, the people and resources needed to help you achieve success. As you learn to consistently utilize this gift of visualization, miracles will begin to occur in your life and circumstances.

As you move forward and set goals, don't worry about how these things will come about, simply move forward in faith, keep your visions clear, work hard every day with a sense of purpose and enjoy the miracles as they occur in your life.

Be Expectant of the Extraordinary

"You may not always get what you want, but you will almost always get what you expect." This quote demonstrates well why this section is a key to success. Dr. Denis Waitley recognized that the most outward, recognizable characteristic of a successful person is positive self-expectation. Earl Nightingale stated that winners are never surprised when they win, simply because that was their expectation from the outset. Positive thinking or optimism is an empowering state of mind or attitude that will bring about extraordinary results. Dozens of research studies in psychology and education have proven that we will produce precisely what we expect from ourselves and what others feel we are capable of producing.

As we raise our own self-expectancy and self-image, others will raise their expectancy and respect for us. The old adage that our attitude will determine our altitude has certainly been born out. Psychologists have proven through research that the 80 percent of the total population that do not perform up to their capability typically have a poor self-image and low self-expectations. The research has shown that the major difference between those 80 percent and the 20 percent of successful to ultra-successful people is purely and simply attitude. It is vital, then, to be expectant of the extraordinary from ourselves. Every human being is unique and possesses the gifts and talents to be extraordinary at something—the key is to seek that special purpose in life, and then be expectant of the extraordinary and it will most assuredly happen. Dr. Norman

Vincent Peale sums it up in his classic book, *The Power of Positive Thinking,* when he concludes that, "If you think positive thoughts, you purely and simply will get positive results."

Learn the Art of Motivation

Learning and understanding the art of motivation is one of the critical keys in the steps to success. One of the most empowering factors for motivation in goal setting is to list the reasons for desiring to achieve each goal. Remember, without specific reasons for achieving your goals, you are much less likely to accomplish them. When we learn to utilize and respond positively to feedback, we will employ the art of motivation. Two kinds of feedback provide awareness and empowerment that move us toward our life goals.

The first, internal feedback, is the inner emotional feeling or response as we perceive an action, a thought, or a circumstance. This inner response can come from our own thought and actions, successes or failures, or from the observation of statements, actions, or circumstances of others. These feelings and perceptions can range anywhere from exhilaration to depression to any place in between. Whether positive or negative, we can learn from this internal feedback, take the invaluable data, program it into our library of information, and utilize it for future reference, either to avoid the pitfalls of failure or for the accomplishment of successes.

The second, external feedback, comes from others through direct responses, acceptance, rejection, opinions, evaluations, constructive criticisms, etc. Once again, whether positive or negative, it can be invaluable in moving us toward our successes while assisting us in avoiding pitfalls.

Learn the Art of Communication

Every successful person considers himself or herself an ongoing self-improvement project. A major part of this self-improvement is the art of communication. Those who master it in this high-tech world will have access to success and the universe. The wise individual and successful person will master the skills of listening, speaking, and writing. The ability to watch, read, hear, and interpret the thoughts, ideas, needs, and desires of others is critical in the processes and procedures of success. Equally important is developing the ability to convey your thoughts, ideas, needs, and desires to others effectively.

Employ the Power of a Thankful Heart

Developing an attitude of gratitude is one of the most powerful things you can do in your life to bring about positive changes that will bring success and generate feelings of peace, contentment and enthusiasm. When you express gratitude for all parts of your life daily, you begin to see your life and self in a different, very positive perspective. When you become more thankful for what you have and what has happened, you will begin to excitedly look forward to the future and what will happen.

Become A Serious Student

Knowledge is power. Successful people are very much aware of this basic truth. So, if you are really serious about success, then become a serious student and begin to tap the treasury of knowledge, if you have not already done so. Go to the library, read the books, listen to the tapes, go to classes, attend the seminars, get on the internet, etc. The idea is to learn, learn, learn.

Discover the Magic of Giving

Mankind has forever searched for purpose and the reason for existing. The most frequent conclusion reached for man's existence is that we are here to build up, encourage, and serve our fellow man. Those who have discovered and employed this secret to life have achieved man's most desired commodity: inner peace.

When we serve, we simply give. Giving is one of the magical keys to success and life. Giving causes us to grow and achieve a maturity and wholeness that can be achieved in no other way. It has been proven time and again that we can only receive back that which we give away. Giving to others has a powerful built-in healing ability.

Further Reading

I would like to recommend some books in the area of the mind-body connection and the role it can play in effectively regaining optimal health. My recommendations follow below:

- *The Healer Within,* by Stephen Locke, M.D.: Dr. Locke gives a thorough view of the science of psychoneuroimmunology that is very detailed, but is very readable, and very understandable. This book also includes a lengthy appendix of organizations and resources to turn to for further help.

- *Nutrition and Your Immune System,* by Carlson Wade: This book gives you a good understanding of your immune system including a definition, how it works, and discussion of the diseases that are caused by a weakened immune system.
- *Love, Medicine, and Miracles,* by Berney S. Siegel, M.D.: This is another excellent book in which Dr. Siegel explores the common physiological characteristics of his patients who have recovered from serious illnesses such as cancer.
- *The Success Journal,* by Dr. Joe M. Elrod: A complete success system developed to assist you in achieving your life goals. Contains a life balance scale and a daily, weekly, monthly success tracking system. Refer to the Resource List for information on how to order your copy.

Personal Commitment Statement

Acknowledging that only I can define success for myself, I, _____, agree that my success plan can be designed only by me and fulfilled by my consistent, determined actions. I agree that commitment to my plan is the first step in achieving the success that I desire. I will use this plan to set my goals, and I will use this plan to track my success.

I recognize that to reach my goals and to realize my fullest potential, I must strive consistently with a positive mental attitude. I promise to daily work at improving my skills and increasing my knowledge so as to achieve the realization of getting well and becoming all that I was intended to be. Finally, I will commit to following this plan.

_____   _____
Date   Signature

LIFE RATING SCALE

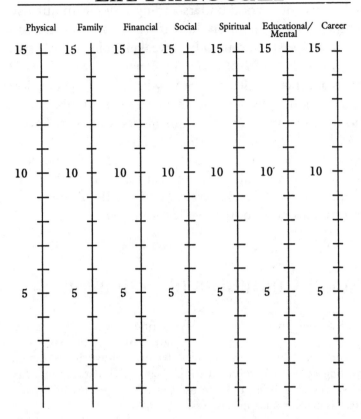

Physical	Family	Financial	Social	Spiritual	Educational/ Mental	Career

Rate each item from one (1) to three (3), with 1 not being well balanced and 3 being very well balanced. There is a possible 15 subtotal under each area of life with a possible 105 as a grand total. Score the five items under each area of life, compute your subtotal and indicate your score on the scale (e.g. your scores in the physical area are 2,1,3,2,3, giving a subtotal of 11; now mark the column at the 11 mark). Once you have scored each area of life, and you have indicated where your score falls on the chart, then connect the scores with a line. This will give you a visual profile of your life balance. Finally, add your subtotals to get your grand total and rate yourself on the following scale:

30-50 = Not Well Balanced
51-80 = Getting There (Average)
81-105 = Very Well Balanced

CHAPTER 5

The Nutrition Factor

"Let your food be your medicine, let your medicine be your food."
Hippocrates

Nutrition is a critical factor in the onset of and treatment of fibromyalgia. The foods that we eat can either strengthen or weaken our immune systems making us more or less vulnerable to the symptoms of disease such as fibromyalgia. Following the nutritional guidelines in this chapter will enhance your immune system and greatly lower your chances for fibromyalgia as well as heart disease, cancer, arthritis, diabetes, and stroke. I will also discuss foods that may help or hinder fibromyalgia along with the essentials of a good nutrition program including supplements such as vitamins, minerals, and antioxidants. Finally, I will discuss the effect of various medications concerning nutritional needs, along with key essentials of healthy weight control.

Balance is the Key in Nutrition

Your body needs a variety of nutrients in order to function at peak performance, including fats, carbohydrates, protein, fiber, vitamins, minerals, and phytochemicals. In fact, the body needs 90 nutrients daily, including 60 minerals, 16 vitamins, 12 essential amino acids, and 3 essential fatty acids. A key to remember here is when treating fibromyalgia or any other chronic condition it is essential to eat a variety of food amounts and combinations. If one continuously eats the same foods over and over, one may miss out on many of the important building blocks in a healthful regimen.

The lower quality of our foods today enhance the weakening of our immune systems and increase the potential for chronic conditions such as fibromyalgia. In the past more plants were organically grown and soils were much richer in a wider range of essential minerals. In today's commercial agriculture, healthy plants are artificially created by the use of herbicides, fungicides, fertilizers, and pesticides. When chemicals are sprayed on plants essential soil microbes are killed that help plants, absorb minerals into their root systems. So then, it is most difficult to absorb adequate levels of the essential nutrients when they are simply not available in the soil. Therefore, we should seek out more foods that are grown organically and that possess more of the vitamins and minerals without all the added chemicals (Weintraub, 1997).

The Value of Antioxidants

Scientific researchers are consistently establishing the fact that a healthful nutritional regimen is one of the key components in safeguarding our health against chronic conditions such as fibromyalgia. One of the most widely accepted theories is that disease and debilitation of the body is basically caused by unstable molecules called free radicals that rampage through the body, attacking healthy cells and destroying healthy tissue. A free radical is defined as a molecule that's missing an electron because of breathing polluted air, metabolizing food substances in the body, consuming unhealthy food additives, etc. These molecules that are missing electrons are not happy until they take a bite out of a healthy cell, damaging it, and replacing the electron that is missing (Bucci 1994). Excessive and nonbuffered free radicals are now thought to be the basic underlying cause of all diseases, including cancer, heart disease, diabetes, arthritis, and degenerative diseases and chronic conditions such as fibromyalgia.

The good news is that the bufferers for free radicals and good health are found in the form of antioxidants. Antioxidants derive their name because they serve as antidotes to one of the free radicals most commonly found in the body—oxygen. Antioxidants buffer or stabilize the free radicals preventing them from attacking and damaging other body tissues (Nierenberg, 1996). The following discussion will reveal where we find many of these antioxidants in a healthful nutrition program in the form of vitamins, minerals, carotenoids, bioflavonoids, and phytonutrients.

EATING TO COMBAT FIBROMYALGIA

The most healthful eating patterns are to eat four to five, even six times daily, enjoying snacks (healthful snacks) for energy and nutrition. Never skip breakfast. Most unhealthy and/or overweight people develop the habit of skipping breakfast. Always eat the traditional breakfast, lunch, and dinner meals with a couple or three healthy snacks in between. The following are a few suggestions for eating throughout the day:

- Eat every few hours to maintain energy, to avoid getting too hungry, and to keep metabolism at its maximum.
- Nutritious snacks should be stashed both at work and at home (i.e., raw fruits and vegetables, vegetable and fruit juices, dried fruit, whole grain crackers, bagels, unsalted nuts, pretzels, and popcorn without butter.
- When concerned about late morning and late afternoon snacks that might ruin your appetite for the good meal, choose a piece of fruit, whole grain bread sticks or crackers, or nibble on raw vegetables. If you will work toward eliminating sugared cereals, soft drinks, candy, cookies, food additives and preservatives, you can quickly enhance the turn-around of the fibromyalgia symptoms, especially pain and the inability to sleep more soundly.
- Remember that everyone should eat a wide variety of foods focusing on the 90 nutrients needed daily. Most people will benefit from eating more fresh fruits and vegetables, seeds, nuts, cereals and whole grains. These foods and others to be listed later provide the necessary increased fiber and fluid, the higher quality fats, the complex carbohydrates, the necessary proteins, and the vitamins and minerals necessary for optimal health and for combating fibromyalgia symptoms. The following guidelines will outline some healthful suggestions for a balanced nutritional program:
- Complex carbohydrates should make up approximately 60-70 percent of your calories. Carbohydrates are, no doubt, one of the most important foods as they provide most of

the fuel for the moving body and the working, healing muscles. (And remember that the fibromyalgia condition is primarily located within the muscles and connective tissues.) Remember that energy is one of the primary problems with the fibromyalgia patient and that complex carbohydrates taken in on a daily basis will increase and maintain a high energy level.

- Fat should make up approximately 20 percent of your calories. Although fat has been tabbed as the culprit in heart disease and obesity, it is a necessary component in a healthful nutrition regimen. It is essential here to read your labels and get most of your fat from healthy sources such as polyunsaturates and monounsaturates such as canola, olive, safflower, peanut, and corn oils.
- Protein is also essential for balance, however, it should make up only 10-15 percent of your calories. Include protein from beans, legumes, nuts, other vegetables along with chicken, turkey, tuna, and fish. Utilize these sources of protein, rather than red meats which, in my opinion and as a result of research, is a detriment to the fibromyalgia victim.
- Avoid junk or fast foods and keep your diet very high in vegetable proteins. A very good suggestion would be to have a green salad and a portion of some type of beans everyday.
- By all means use purified water, ideally 8-10 eight-ounce glasses per day. A water purification system in the home is highly desirable to provide the pure water for cooking and drinking.
- It is essential to remove as many artificial food additives and chemicals as possible from your nutritional program.
- Avoid caffeine, sugar, and any unnecessary drugs not prescribed by your physician.
- Avoid refined and processed foods as much as possible, especially foods that are canned or boxed as they always

have more additives. Fresh foods always have fewer additives and sometimes will have none at all.(Elrod, 1996)

THE MIRACLE NUTRIENTS

In this segment I will discuss some of the better sources of antioxidants, vitamins, minerals, enzymes, and other supplemental miracle nutrients. The more powerful antioxidant vitamins are beta carotene, vitamin C, vitamin E, and vitamin B6. Some of the trace minerals that serve as powerful antioxidants are selenium, zinc, manganese, magnesium, boron, and chromium. Some other powerful antioxidant and immune boosting nutrients are coenzyme Q-10, proanthocianidins, or pycnogenol (from grape seeds), rice bran extract, curcumin, and garlic. The foods and supplements that can provide the above miracle nutrients are very powerful weapons for fighting against and buffering free radicals and the damage they can deliver. The following are some excellent sources for the miracle nutrients in the suggested above areas:

- *Beta Carotene*: There are dozens of carotinoids of which beta carotene is one in the plant form of vitamin A. The better sources of carotinoids are yellow and orange fruits and vegetables such as carrots, cantaloupe, sweet potatoes, pumpkin, apricots, and melons such as mango, papaya, peaches and winter squash. The dark green leafy vegetables are another excellent source of beta carotene. Examples are collard greens, parsley, spinach, broccoli, and other leafy greens.
- *Vitamin C:* This is one of the more powerful antioxidants and the major sources are fresh fruits such as grapefruit,

strawberries, bananas, cantaloupe, papaya, kiwi, mango, raspberries, pineapple, and tomatoes, as well as fresh vegetables such as cabbage, asparagus, broccoli, Brussels sprouts, collard greens, potatoes, and red peppers. Vitamin C is highly heat sensitive and easily destroyed by refining or over-processing therefore should be steamed or microwaved for a very short period of time.

- *Vitamin E:* The better sources for this powerful antioxidant are vegetable oils, especially safflower, avocados, nuts, sunflower seeds, wheat germ, whole grain cereals and breads, asparagus, dried prunes, and broccoli.
- *Selenium:* There is much evidence to substantiate that selenium boosts the immune system by protecting cells from the toxic effects of free radicals. Some of the better food sources of selenium are shrimp, sunflower seeds, wheat breads, tuna and salmon.
- *Zinc:* This trace mineral assists in performing many of the vital body functions. For instance, it helps with the absorption of vitamins in the body and helps form skin, nails, and hair, as well as being an essential part of many enzymes involved in metabolism and digestion. Vitamin A must be present for zinc to be properly absorbed in the body. Some excellent sources of zinc are ginseng, chalk, and the herb licorice.
- *Manganese:* A trace mineral essential for the proper functioning of the pituitary gland as well as healthy functioning of the body's other glands. It is essential in the treatment and healing of fibromyalgia in that it is an excellent aid in the utilization of glucose in the process of creating energy and it also helps in the normal functioning of the central nervous system.
- *Magnesium:* This is a very essential part of the enzyme system and is seemingly most important in the rehabilitation from fibromyalgia. Almost 100 percent of the fibromyalgia

victims with which I have worked have exhibited a magnesium deficiency. Another critical function of magnesium is in the absorption of potassium, calcium, phosphorus, the B complex vitamins, as well as vitamins C and E. Magnesium is also essential in ATP (energy) production.

- *Malic Acid:* Another essential ingredient in the energy production process. Critical in lessening the toxic effects of aluminum. When combined with magnesium, malic acid is very effective as a cleansing and healing agent for fibromyalgia and other systemic conditions.

- *Chromium:* This trace mineral is essential for the synthesis of fatty acids and the metabolism of glucose for energy. It is also well known for its ability to increase the efficiency of insulin.

- *Boron:* This trace mineral possesses some antioxidant functions and is very important in maintaining muscular health in that it assists in inhibiting cells from releasing free radicals. Cauliflower and apples are sources of boron.

- *Coenzyme Q-10:* Research studies indicate that this enzyme increases a vital component of the immune system (gamma globulin). Co Q-10 proves valuable in the treatment of fibromyalgia because it is a very important component for enhancing circulation and increasing the energy level.

- *Proanthocyanidins:* One of the potent sources of proanthocyanidins is pycnogenol from a grape seed extract. The pycnogenol from grape seed is a very powerful antioxidant and is 50 times stronger than vitamin E. It is also very efficient in boosting the immune system and assisting in the treatment of fibromyalgia.

- *Rice Bran Extract:* There are three polyphenols from the tocotryonols of rice bran that are 6,000 times stronger than vitamin E.

- *Glucosamine:* The key substance that determines how many proteoglycan (water holding) molecules are formed in cartilage. Glucosamine has been found to be very effective for improvement in arthritic conditions. Also, in a study conducted by the Vulvodynia Project, it was used to effectively reduce sensitivity and pain in soft tissue areas of fibromyalgia patients.

• *Chrondroitin Sulfate:* Naturally occurring substances that inhibit the enzymes that can degrade cartilage while helping to attract fluid to the proteoglycan molecules.

As mentioned earlier, it is generally best to get vitamins, minerals, antioxidants, and the nutrients the body needs from fresh whole foods (ideally organic foods) rather than supplements. However, it is common knowledge that the proper amounts of vitamins, minerals, and nutrients are very difficult to acquire from foods because of depleted soils and the use of chemicals in the form of pesticides and insecticides. In order to get all of the necessary nutrients in today's world it is absolutely essential that supplements are taken, especially when treating chronic conditions such as fibromyalgia.

Is nutritional supplementation really necessary for healing and health? The answer is an unequivocal "yes." A well controlled study performed at the Shriner's Burn Trauma Center at the University of Cincinnati Medical School demonstrated conclusively that burn trauma victims of children's age faired far better when given extra nutritional supplementation over and above the normal "well-balanced diet" generally prescribed by practitioners. One hundred percent of the children receiving the extra supplementation lived, whereas tragically 44 percent of the children who were given the regular traditional medically and so-called balanced diet alone died. The scientists stated that, "To our knowledge this is the first controlled study to demonstrate what has been suspected and accepted for some time, that nutritional intervention improves survival."

Vitamins/Minerals/Nutrients Maximum Daily Dosage

The following is a table of the essential nutrients and recommended dosages for fibromyalgia and related systemic conditions:

ESSENTIAL NUTRIENT	RECOMMENDED DOSAGE
Beta Carotene	25,000 IUs
Vitamin C	1,000-3,000 milligrams
Vitamin E	400-800 IUs
Selenium	200 micrograms
Zinc	30 milligrams
Magnesium	400 milligrams
Manganese	10 milligrams
Chromium	200 micrograms
Coenzyme Q-10	50 milligrams
Pycnogenol	50 milligrams
Rice Bran Extract	50 milligrams
Boron	3 milligrams
Malic Acid/Magnesium Hydroxine (taken in 4-6 doses)	2,000-4,000 milligrams
Glucosamine	1,000-1,500 milligrams
Chondroitin Sulfate	800-1,200 milligrams

MUSCLE/CONNECTIVE TISSUE AND BIOFLAVONOIDS

There are literally thousands of different types of bioflavonoids. They are found in virtually all plant foods and are essential for healthy capillary walls, the metabolism of vitamin C, and enhancing the utilization of other essential nutrients. The bioflavonoids aid fibromyalgia victims by:

- Enhancing the strength of collagen in connective tissue
- Strengthening muscle fiber
- Buffering free radical damage
- Enhancing the functioning ability of muscle fiber
- Enhancing the energy production process
- Enhancing the utilization of other nutrients in the body

Some excellent sources of bioflavonoids are fresh fruits and vegetables, seeds, nuts, legumes, whole grains, citrus fruits, onions, berries, green tea, and especially fruits that contain a pit (such as plums and cherries). There are also rosehip bioflavonoids as well as citrus bioflavonoids such as catechin, hesperidin, rutin, quercetin, milk thistle seed extract, gingko biloba extracts, pycnogenol (from grape seed extract), and rice bran extract (Carper, 1995).

Maintaining a Healthy Weight

Being overweight is directly related to at least sixty-seven other diseases; specifically high blood pressure, heart disease, diabetes, secondary osteoarthritis, fibromyalgia, stress and depression. By employing a good weight maintenance program or by reducing your weight (if you are overweight) you can greatly improve the symptoms of fibromyalgia. Remember a healthy weight is one of the major components of your health and wellness program during the healing and recovery process.

Following highly restrictive diets or crash diets that are based on a limited number of foods are not healthy physiologically and basically do not work in the long run. On many of these diets you will almost always lose weight initially, and sometimes a great deal of weight in the first week or two, and feel that you are beginning a program on which you are highly successful. However, again, these programs are not healthy and do not work for the long term. Research studies show that people who go on the stringent or highly restrictive diets usually lose weight but then gain it over and over again. These people normally become fatter over the long haul and also have a higher mortality rate than those who remain at a constant weight on a very healthy weight maintenance program. This is why it is very important to make a lifestyle change where you are adhering to healthful lifestyle prescription on a daily basis. This can really make the difference for health and longevity. A key is to choose a very easy, flexible, sensible nutrition plan that does not call for special shopping or tedious calorie counting, such as the plan provided for you here.

The following are a few guidelines to assist you along the way on your sensible, flexible and healthful lifetime weight management program. The individuals who have lost weight successfully and kept it off have generally utilized the following guidelines:

- *Make a commitment to change.* Without a firm commitment, chances for change are not very likely. This must be your goal to improve your health, lose weight, and reduce the symptoms of your fibromyalgia. If this is the goal of your physician or a family member, but not your own, then it's not likely that you'll be successful.
- *Plan ahead and be organized.* Do not eat sporadically and/or automatically. Do not prepare or serve more than can be eaten. Those who are successful with their programs prepare in advance for well balanced meals at home and for

upcoming events, even taking their own food to a function if necessary. Always arrange a schedule so that you have time for your exercise sessions and meals. These are two of the most important events of the day. Never skip meals, especially breakfast.

- *Set challenging but realistic goals.* Goal-oriented people are usually successful with most of their efforts. However, you must be realistic with your goals, not to lose too much weight in too short a period of time and not to have a goal for weight that is most unrealistic for your height and body type. A healthy weight loss rate is no more than two pounds per week.

- *Prepare wisely.* Prepare healthfully by boiling, baking, and steaming. It is very important to include at least 20 percent fat in your meals but be sure that you are getting the proper amount and the healthy fats (see the following 21 Day Detoxification Program).

- *Keep busy and productive.* Do not use eating to occupy leisure time. Always eat the four to five meals per day, but do not break your rule and use eating to occupy leisure time. Be sure that you're exercising regularly, getting the proper kinds of exercise every day. Keeping your body moving continuously raises and keeps your metabolic rate up, burning calories all day, even hours after your exercise session and even when you are resting. The regular exercise will increase your lean body tissue and decrease your body fat tissue, and this raises your metabolic rate in that lean tissue requires calories whereas fat does not.

- *Beware of social binges.* Eat wisely at functions and avoid refrigerator raids. If you use alcohol at all, and especially at social functions, be sure that it's used in great moderation. This is very important to your weight maintenance program and most vital to your healing process from your fibromyalgia.

- *Monitor progress and reward accomplishments.* Keep track of percent body fat and loss in inches and pounds during reasonable periods. Do not be concerned with weighing and measuring on a daily basis. Remember that people who are successful at losing and maintaining their weight and improving their health do not follow stringent or crash diets nor do they burden themselves with calorie counting. Focus on total health and wellness and getting well. Do not be so concerned with numbers on the scale nor how much farther you can walk each day. Simply allow those things to happen naturally as you are getting healthier, feeling better, and getting well.

- *Practice effective stress management techniques.* Learn deep breathing and muscle relaxation exercises. If you need, go to a professional to learn these procedures in a very efficient manner. Be organized and efficient with time, as this is one of the major stress relievers. Remember to get 7-8 hours of sleep every night, always retiring at the same time establishing a habit pattern to enhance the effective and efficient sleep pattern. Include a minimum of two and possibly three fifteen-minute relaxation sessions on a daily basis. This will add tremendously to your health and vitality and to your recovery.

- *Develop a positive success attitude.* Concentrate on succeeding and not negative past habit patterns or failure. Avoid negative environments and negative people who will not be supportive. Focus on why you have developed poor eating habits and what those poor habits were, times of day you were eating, what you were eating and how you were preparing. Finally, make a conscious effort to change those behaviors.

Dr. Elrod's 21-Day Detoxification Program

Detoxification is the process of body and/or cell cleansing through purging of toxic buildup resultant of a combination of poor diet, ingestion of abusive substances, and stress. An abusive lifestyle, including the ingestion of excessive fat, junk foods, nicotine, caffeine, excessive alcohol, other drugs, a lack of rest, and undue stress will eventually create a toxic buildup within the body and begin to break down the immune system.

I have designed the following dietary guidelines to promote body cleansing as a first step back toward health and wellness, and as a new beginning for strengthening the immune system. The body doesn't like shock, so ideally a ten-day tapering period of gradually reducing sugar, fat, caffeine, etc., is advised before beginning the 21-day detoxification program. The ten-day tapering period is important in assisting the body to adjust and to insure success with the total program. As you can see, within a 30-day period, the cleansing (detoxification) process will be complete and you will be on your way back to a happy, healthy, and successful lifestyle.

THINGS TO EMPHASIZE

These are areas that one should emphasize in nutritional habits for achieving a successful detoxification program:

1. Increase high fiber foods, gradually: vegetables, fresh fruits, whole grains, seeds and nuts, and legumes. Be sure to include peaches, strawberries, potatoes, spinach, tomatoes, wheat and bran cereals, whole wheat bread, rice, and popcorn.
2. Increase raw fruits and vegetables to 50 percent of your diet. Be sure to include cucumbers, radishes, grapefruit,

apples, carrots, cantaloupe, red bell peppers, and green leafy vegetables.

3. Drink pure water (10 to 12 glasses a day).
4. Eat moderately and more deliberately. No television or reading while eating; emphasize family conversation.
5. Eat a maximum of 1500 calories per day for 21 days.
6. Employ the thankful heart attitude for your food and health.
7. Visualization: For each of these 21 days, visualize yourself getting well while maintaining your ideal body weight and shape.

THINGS TO AVOID

The following are foods and other nutritional to avoid in order to achieve a successful detoxification program:

1. High fat dairy products
2. White sugar and white flour
3. Fried foods
4. Preservatives, junk food, and salt
5. Red meat (especially salt-cured, smoked, nitrate-cured foods like bacon, pepperoni, etc.) and chicken (which is a high-fat food)
6. Coffee and caffeinated teas
7. Colas, soda pop, and carbonated beverages
8. Liquids with your meals (Drink acceptable liquids one hour before and two hours after meals. Drinking during meals dilutes hydrochloric acid.)
9. Alcoholic beverages
10. All forms of tobacco
11. Prolonged periods in direct sun rays (Protect yourself with at least 15 SPF sunscreen; wear long sleeves and hat between 11 a.m. and 3 p.m.)
12. NutraSweet and saccharine.

Note: Consume 25 percent of total calories at breakfast. Consume 50 percent of total calories at lunch. Consume 25 percent of total calories at dinner. (Do not count the two or three healthful snacks.)

NOW WHAT AFTER 21 DAYS?

After you have successfully completed your detoxification and immune system strengthening program, you will not necessarily continue with the above stringent nutritional prgram. However, you will want to continue a prudent, healthful program to keep you on track for a happy, healthy, successful life. For example, you will want to adhere to the following healthful eating guidelines:

- Continue high fiber content in diet (fruits, vegetables, whole grains and cereals).
- Choose whole wheat breads, bran cereals, rice, and pasta.
- Consume legumes (beans, lentils and nuts).
- Use low-fat dairy products.
- Limit or eliminate red meats.
- Eat chicken or turkey (no skin), tuna and fish in place of red meat.
- Emphasize fruits, vegetables, and salads (low-cal dressings).
- Ingest omega-3 fatty acids (fish oils).
- Drink purified water (10 to 12 glasses per day).
- Increase calories back to normal maintenance levels for active individuals (1800 to 2400 for females, 2400 to 3000 for males) once desired weight has been achieved.

PROBLEMS WITH ADDITIVES, METALS AND OTHER TOXINS

There is a strong link between heavy toxic metals, food additives, other toxins and poor nutrition. Toxic metals are commonly found in commercially processed foods that typically contain food colorings and additives. Pesticides, herbicides and other agricultural chemicals still present us with numerous nutritional issues. The following sections address the problems with metals, food additives and other toxins commonly consumed in the average diet (For more complete information on this topic, see Dr. Skye Weintraub's title, *Natural Treatments for ADD and Hyperactivity*, 1997).

Metals

Let's take a look at some of the metals commonly found in the body and that become toxic and cause degenerative and serious health problems. There are treatment plans available for treating and removing toxic metals from the body and there are also naturopathic health practitioners who do toxicity testing.

MERCURY

Mercury amalgam tooth fillings are one of the primary sources for mercury leakage into the body. Some of the other common places to find mercury include processed foods, drinking water, pesticides, fertilizers, mascara, floor waxes, body powder, adhesives, wood preservatives, batteries, and air conditioning filters. Finally, mercury is second only to cadmium as being the most toxic heavy metal on earth.

LEAD

Lead is linked to a number of neurological and psychological disturbances. Lead affects brain function because of its neurotoxic effects. Our drinking water appears to be one of the more prominent sources from which we accumulate lead into the body.

One precaution is to have your water supply tested for high lead levels. The use of lead-based solders in modern copper plumbing systems increases the intake of lead through the very water we drink. Filter your home water supply with a filter that will remove heavy metals.

Always wash your fruits and vegetables in filtered water before use, not tap water. If possible buy your produce from farms and areas that have low air pollution. Do not use any imported canned food as the cans are often lead lined.

COPPER

Stress from fibromyalgia can lead to copper toxicity. When the adrenal glands function properly, they produce a copper bonding protein, therefore, stress can deplete zinc from body tissue which taxes the adrenal glands. People who consume large amounts of soda pop, junk foods, and other empty-calorie foods are much more prone to copper toxicity problems. This can help to lower the immune system and cause the individual to have recurrent infections more readily.

MANGANESE

Excessive toxic levels of manganese are toxic to the brain's neurons. There is typically emotional instability associated with manganese overload, such as easy laughter or crying, muscular weakness, slowed speech, and impaired equilibrium.

CADMIUM

Cadmium levels are typically higher in people that eat excessive amounts of carbohydrates. This suggests that the consumption of fast or refined foods that are low in nutrients increases the body's cadmium levels. Adequate zinc intake may help protect against the adverse effects of cadmium. Once cadmium is in the body it is very difficult to remove because of its seventeen to thirty year lifespan. Elimination of cadmium from the body is generally accomplished through nutritional therapy (See the 21-day Detoxification Program).

Cigarettes are one of the major sources of cadmium in our society. Zinc, used for galvanizing iron, can contain up to two percent cadmium and this is one reason our tap water is normally contaminated.

ALUMINUM

High levels of aluminum affect the central nervous system and is suspected to be intricately involved in the problems of fibromyalgia sufferers. Some of the primary sources of aluminum are in the very aluminum cookware used in homes, as well as aluminum foil in which we frequently store food. Aluminum is also found in antacids, bleached flour, and coffee. Deficiencies of magnesium and calcium may greatly increase the toxic effects of aluminum in the body.

Food Additives

About 70-80 percent of the foods we consume undergo some degree of refinement or chemical alteration. The Department of National Health and Welfare explains that additives are usually chemical in nature and do not include seasonings, spices, or natural flavorings. Consumers in

America use approximately 100 million pounds of food additives per year. The FDA in the United States allows more than 10,000 food and chemical additives in our food supply. The average American consumes between 10 and 15 pounds of salt and additives per year (Gans, 1991).

There are two categories of food additives: those that make food more pleasant to the eyes and more appealing to the tastebuds and, secondly, those that prevent food from spoiling or that increase their shelf life.

BHT

Butylated hydroxytoluene (BHT) retards rancidity in frozen and fresh pork sausage and freeze-dried meats. The base product used in shortenings and animal fats contains BHT and is also the base product for chewing gum. Enlargement of the liver and allergic reactions are two of the adverse effects that have been exhibited from the use of BHT.

BHA

Butylated hydroxyanisole (BHA) is also an antioxidant and effects liver and kidney function within human beings. BHA has been associated with behavior problems in children and is commonly used as a preservative in a wide variety of products like baked goods, candy, chewing gum, soup bases, breakfast cereals, shortening, dry mixes for desserts, potatoes, potato flakes, and ice cream.

CAFFEINE

Caffeine can affect blood sugar release and uptake by the liver and is a central nervous system, heart, and respiratory stimulant. Caffeine is a natural ingredient in tea, coffee, and cola and some of its ill effects are irregular heartbeat, ear noises, insomnia, irritability and nervousness.

101

ASPARTAME

Equal and NutraSweet are the actual marketed names of aspartame. Aspartame intensifies the taste of sweeteners and flavors and is about 200 times sweeter than sucrose. Recent research studies have discovered that memory loss attributed to diabetes is caused by aspartame. Large amounts consumed over time will upset neurotransmitter balance as well as the amino acid balance within the body.

MSG

Canned tuna, snack foods, and soups and a large percentage of prepared foods now found on grocery store shelves contain MSG. Monosodium glutamate is now the most common flavor enhancer added to foods on the market.

It is very difficult to identify MSG within products from labels because the manufacturers are not required to call it MSG on the label. MSG is very frequently disguised with such names as sodium caseinate, hydrolyzed yeast, hydrolyzed vegetable protein, and autolyzed yeast. Some of the other names used to disguise MSG are textured protein, hydrolyzed protein, yeast food, calcium caseinate, natural chicken or turkey flavoring, yeast extract, hydrolyzed yeast, natural flavoring, and other spices.

PHOSPHATES

Phosphates attract the trace minerals in foods and then continue to remove them from the body. There are phosphates in cheese, baked goods, carbonated drinks, canned meats, powdered foods, dry cereals, and cola drinks. Phosphates are a preservative that prevent the outward and chemical changes of food including texture, appearance, flavor, and color.

SORBATE

Sorbate is a fungus preventative and preservative used in chocolate syrups, drinks, soda fountain syrups, baked goods, deli salads, cheese cake, fresh fruit cocktail, pie fillings, preserves, and artificially sweetened jellies.

SULFITES

Sulfites are preservatives and bleaching agents found in sliced fruit, beer, ale, and wine. They are commonly found in packaged lemon juice, potatoes, salad dressings, gravies, corn syrup, wine vinegar, avocado dip, and sauces.

Sulfites are primarily used to reduce or prevent discoloration of light colored vegetables and fruits such as dehydrated potatoes and dried apples. Sulfites assist vegetables and fruits to look fresh.

What's Wrong with Sugar?

Empty sugar calories provided from sucrose usually crowd out nutritious foods and they do not provide vitamins, minerals, or fiber. Manufacturers advertise that their sugar products will provide quick energy, but the quick energy is very short-lived because in about twenty minutes or so after consumption an individual will feel cranky, tired, sluggish and sometimes even mildly depressed. If you eat between meal snacks frequently including candy and sugared sodas you are paving the way for poor health and opening the door for systemic conditions such as fibromyalgia.

IS SUGAR ADDICTIVE?

The answer to this question is an certain "yes." Sugar acts very similar to a drug when eaten in large amounts or if consumed daily. Sugar is one of the most damaging and destructive items in our daily diets. It is one of the primary culprits in destroying the ability of the immune system to retain its strength. Some suggested sweeteners that are healthier for those who really desire or need sweeteners are pure maple syrup, rice syrup, molasses, sucanat, honey, date sugar, or stevia (Weintraub, 1996).

COMPARING THE VARIOUS TYPES OF SUGARS

Sugar in any form is very quickly absorbed into the blood stream and provides quick energy for the body. However, remember that sugar, whether it be from sugar cane, sugar beets, or from corn, is completely refined, has no nutritional value, and provides only empty calories. All the sugars are treated the same by the body, converting them all to glucose, whether they are sucrose, fructose, or dextrose. Once converted to glucose, it is circulated through the blood stream as an energy source and stored in the liver and the muscles as fat. Just a note to remember here is that most fruit juices are as much of a sweet as candy, even the unsweetened juices. They are very high in natural sugars and very often have the same harmful effects as pure sugar candy or other sweets.

POWER FOODS

The following are "power" foods that act as bufferers to various diseases and complicated conditions in the body. They can help with cancer, heart disease, diabetes, fibromyalgia, and other systemic conditions.

BRAN CEREAL

Bran cereal is very high in wheat bran and this is one of the best sources of cancer fighting insoluble fiber, the kind of fiber that increases stool bulk and speed. This is a cereal that provides about five grams of fiber per serving.

BROWN RICE

The high fiber rice bran in brown rice possibly can help to lower cholesterol. Brown rice is very high in vitamin B-6 and magnesium. It provides thiamine (which is vital to nerve function), niacin, copper, and zinc. Research studies indicate that vitamin E from brown rice tends to strengthen the immune system and will reduce the risk of heart disease and cataracts.

BROCCOLI

Broccoli contains potassium and chromium which help to stabilize blood sugar. Broccoli is filled with cancer-fighting fiber, vitamin C, beta carotene, bone-building calcium, folic acid, boron, and sulforaphane which helps to detoxify harmful enzymes in the body.

LEAN BEEF

Very lean beef is a super source of zinc, which is an immune system strengthener, and also contains niacin which may help prevent cancerous conditions. Lean beef will also protect against cell damage that can lead to cancer and it also helps to fend off infections.

CABBAGE

There are substances called indols in cabbage that are anti-cancer agents.

CANTALOUPE

Cantaloupe is absolutely packed with vitamin C, fiber, folic acid, potassium, beta carotene, and vitamin B-6.

CARROTS

Scientific studies suggest that one carrot a day may reduce lung cancer risk in ex-smokers. Carrots are also loaded with beta carotene.

BANANAS

Bananas may help to lower blood pressure. They are high in vitamin B6, rich in potassium, and research indicates that they are essential to building a strong immune system.

BEANS

We get much of our fiber from beans, which helps to regulate blood sugar levels, staves off hunger, and also reduces a diabetic's need for insulin. Beans are also thought to lower blood pressure.

APRICOTS

Apricots are loaded with the antioxidants, beta carotene and vitamin C. Researchers have recently established that vitamin C can help prevent cataracts along with reducing the risk of cancers of the mouth, throat, stomach, and pancreas. Apricots are also packed with fiber, and when combined with a low-fat diet, can lessen the risk of colon polyps.

FISH

The essential fatty acids in fish oils have been found to lower triglycerides (blood fats and sugars). High levels of triglycerides are thought to be more harmful to women than men. It is recommended that fish should be eaten three to four times a week. Lake trout, salmon, sardines, anchovies, herring, and blue fish are those that have the most essential fatty acids.

GARLIC

Garlic helps to protect against heart disease and stroke. It might also lower blood pressure and it acts as a natural antibiotic. Research studies suggest that garlic gives many multiple benefits including the fact that it appears to defuse carcinogenic chemicals (e.g. those from cigarettes).

OATS

Oats lower the LDL (bad) cholesterol. Research studies have found that if individuals eat 3 grams of soluble fiber a day, which is about the amount found in three packets of instant oatmeal, one can lower LDL cholesterol by 6 percent within six weeks.

KIWI

Kiwi is a fruit that is literally packed with vitamin C and cancer-fighting fiber.

GINGER

Ginger is a spice and, like many other spices including rosemary, pepper, oregano, and thyme, is a powerful antioxidant.

SKIM MILK

Research studies show that postmenopausal women who take in 150 milligrams of calcium in supplement form reduce their bone loss. Researchers are now convinced that extra calcium can absolutely strengthen the bones and prevent fractures in older adults. Skim milk appears to be one of the best sources of bone-building calcium and riboflavin. Riboflavin is a B vitamin which helps maintain energy.

ORANGE JUICE

All citrus fruits and juices, including orange juice, contain liminoids. These are substances that research studies have shown that can activate detoxifying enzymes in the body which reduce cancer risk. Orange juice is the classic source of vitamin C, and it is recommended that smokers take twice the amount that non-smokers require.

GRAPES

Grapes are an excellent source of boron, a mineral that helps to prevent osteoporosis. Red grape juice also contains resveratrol a phytochemical that may help prevent heart disease by inhibiting the "clumping" of blood cells.

NUTS

We can classify nuts as a heart helper. For example, adults on a low fat diet who ate two ounces of walnuts, five or more times a week, lowered their cholesterol levels by 12 percent.

MANGOS

Mangos are packed with vitamin B-6 and copper, and with the anticancer antioxidants beta carotene and vitamin C. The combination of these antioxidants have been shown in a USDA study to lower blood pressure.

OLIVE OIL

Olive oil is a key component of the healthy Mediterranean diet. Olive oil is the oil richest in monounsaturated fats which have been shown to lower cholesterol.

LENTILS

Lentils provide a bonanza of nutrients and especially the B-complex vitamins. One particular study done by physicians suggest that they protect against heart attacks because they are very high in fiber, protein and minerals, such as iron and immune-boosting copper, manganese, and zinc.

KALE

Kale is packed with fiber, calcium, manganese, vitamin B-6, copper, and potassium. Kale has provided another hope against heart disease helping to reduce the harmful effects of the LDL cholesterol.

PUMPKIN

Pumpkin is particularly high in beta carotene and fiber.

PEARS

Pears provide vitamin C, potassium, boron, and fiber.

SOY PROTEIN

Soy protein is an invaluable power food in that research studies have shown that populations that have a high soy intake have lowered the rates of heart disease, osteoporosis, and breast cancer.

PRUNES

Prunes are a source of bone-saving boron and of the antioxidant vitamins A and E, and they are loaded with fiber.

RED BELL PEPPERS

Red bell peppers are a better anticancer choice than green peppers because they contain added carotenes. Red bell peppers also supply powerful antioxidant properties, and help fight cancer by inhibiting the formation of carcinogenic nitrosamines (formed when you ingest foods containing nitrates such as bacon, sausage, and cured beef).

SPINACH

Spinach provides a powerhouse of antioxidants and is very rich is folic acid.

SUNFLOWER SEEDS

Sunflower seeds are very high in vitamin E which is an antioxidant that fights heart disease, cancer, and cataracts. Sunflower seeds are very similar to nuts in polyunsaturated fat content.

TEA

Worldwide studies have suggested that the chemicals in tea tend to prevent cancer and lower blood cholesterol.

STRAWBERRIES

Strawberries offer more vitamin C and fiber than most other fruits. Strawberries also contain elegiac acid which is a natural cancer fighting chemical.

TOMATOES

Tomatoes contain lycopene, a chemical also found in pink grapefruit which is thought to help prevent some cancers, including prostate cancer. Tomatoes are also an excellent source of vitamins A and C, as well as fiber and potassium.

WHEAT GERM

Wheat germ is an excellent source of many nutrients. Just 1/4 cup will provide as much as 5 grams of fiber as well as almost all of the daily requirements of magnesium, zinc, iron, and the B-complex vitamins. Wheat germ is incredibly rich in manganese and it is also one of the best sources of chromium and vitamin E.

SWEET POTATOES

Sweet potatoes contain almost twice the fiber and much more beta carotene than white and red potatoes.

YOGURT

Yogurt has been proven in research studies to prevent allergies and colds. Researchers at the University of California at Davis found that people who ate an eight-ounce carton of yogurt with live cultures (specifically lactobacillus, bulgaricus, and streptococcus thermophilous) daily had 25 percent fewer colds and almost 10 times fewer allergy symptoms than those eating the same amount of yogurt with "killed" cultures. Yogurt is a great source of calcium as well. Other research studies have also borne out that yogurt is linked to lowering cholesterol. An individual looking for the better yogurt should look for live cultures listed on the containers.

WHOLE WHEAT FOODS

All whole wheat foods including pasta are very rich in vitamin B6, fiber, and manganese. Whole wheat bread for instance contains triple the fiber of white bread. Everyone needs extra B6 as we age to keep our immune systems strong.

Tracking what you eat, when you eat, the supplements you take, etc., can be beneficial in taking full advantage of your nutritional plan. To help you do this, we have provided a log sheet where you can note your nutritional intake (as well as your exercising, mental activities, and other information) on a daily basis. See the "Daily Log" in Appendix A.

CHAPTER 6

The Exercise Prescription

The right kind of regular exercise is now highly recommended for fibromyalgia sufferers to recover and maintain their health. In fact, regular lifetime exercise helps guard against a host of other health problems such as obesity, diabetes, high blood pressure, and heart disease. It is a proven fact that a lifestyle without exercise is second only to smoking as the most common cause of death in the United States. At one time it was thought that exercise exacerbated the condition of fibromyalgia, but we now know that regular and appropriate exercise is an excellent means of assisting the muscles to become healthy and vibrant.

Exercise is one of the key components in the health and healing regimen for those with existing fibromyalgia. Exercise improves the muscle tone as it increases the nourishing flow of blood into the tissues. It improves flexibility, increases the healing endorphins in the immune system, enhances the production of T-cells that are highly effective in the efficient autoimmune system, and stimulates the secretion of seratonin and the growth hormone. In fact, the right exercises are essential to weight control, reducing pain, and increasing the mobility of the fibromyalgia patient. In the *Journal of Hematology* in 1989 it was reported that the pain in fibromyalgia is related to microtrauma in deconditioned muscles and that exercise works by conditioning these muscles. Also, in a controlled study of the effects of a cardiovascular training program, daily gentle low-impact aerobic exercise was of benefit to fibromyalgia symptoms (McCain 1988). Another outstanding benefit of exercise to the fibromyalgia patient is the improved health of the supportive structures and joints. At one time we thought that exercise actually caused arthritis; however, we now know that regular exercise is an excellent means of aiding in keeping joints healthy.

The old theory that high-impact exercise such as running and high-impact aerobics could wear out joints has been disproved (Fries, 1994). In fact, it has been further proven and documented that regular exercise is strong protection against osteoarthritis (Bunning and Materson, 1991). When you move a joint, as you do in weight resistance exercise or stretching, the nutrient rich synovial fluid in the cartilage is squeezed out, eliminating some of the waste and buffering free radicals just as if the cartilage were a soggy sponge. Consequently, when that pressure is released the fluid rushes back into the cartilage, nourishing it and keeping it moist and healthy. The movement of fluid in the cartilage is critical to the health of the cartilage, for without it the cartilage becomes thin and dry and therefore more susceptible to deterioration and damage. For this reason exercise is an outstanding medicine for osteoarthritis. It keeps the nourishing fluid flowing into the afflicted joint and reduces pressure on the joint by strengthening support structures. As one can see, having healthier joints and stronger support structures around the musculature is a tremendous benefit to the fibromyalgia patient. One can also readily see that the right exercise can help to reduce pain and increase the mobility of the fibromyalgia patient.

The Critical Nature of Exercise

The human body is marvelously designed with muscles and joints acting as levers and pulleys to perform an incredible array of activities. However, when we are ill or injured we have a natural tendency to slow down and stop our normal activities in favor of rest. Sometimes that is definitely the wisest decision, especially if there is a severe back injury or if fever is involved with an illness. However, when we stop moving, the unused muscle and bone will atrophy or waste away. This is exactly what happens to fibromyalgia sufferers who stop normal activities and cut back on the amount of movement and exercise they are getting. They tend to lose muscle tone and strength, and flexibility becomes limited. As a result, the fibromyalgia symptoms progress more rapidly.

Although diet and nutritional supplements help to rebuild and keep the body strong, it is very important to continue exercise to keep the muscles healthy and flexible. Exercise in many different forms, whether it be calisthenics, stretching, weight resistance, walking, swimming, or cycling, is now known to be effective as a most important part of the treatment and healing regimen for fibromyalgia. Exercise fights the debilitating effects of fibromyalgia in the following important ways (Elrod, 1996):

• *Exercise strengthens connective tissue (ligaments and tendons) while enhancing muscle tone.* Strong, well-toned and healthy muscles, tendons, and ligaments can support the body and the body's movement much more efficiently and ward off pain.

- *Exercise increases the flexibility and/or range of motion of muscle tissue.* Highly flexible or pliable muscles make movement much more efficient and pleasant while helping to prevent strains, pulls, and tears. Very simple functions such as stooping, sitting, walking, and exercising become much easier to perform and much more pleasant. When muscles, ligaments, and tendons become more resilient, this means that stiffness will be reduced. Remember that early morning stiffness is one of the major problems and symptoms of fibromyalgia. The resiliency and flexibility that come from exercise also improve the overall muscle and joint function, lessening pain and releasing pent up tensions to aid in the relief of stress.

- *Exercise increases blood flow to the muscles.* An increased blood flow to the muscle tissue enhances the transport of oxygen and nutrients to the muscle fiber, helping to restore and maintain the health of the muscle tissue. We know that people with fibromyalgia do have slightly less blood flow to the muscles which probably contributes to the pain associated with fibromyalgia. Exercise helps reduce this problem.

- *Exercise increases the body's supply of endorphins.* Endorphins released by the hypothalamus are the body's own morphine-like substance, healing and uplifting with a natural pain-relieving and sleep-deepening effect. Neurologist Norman Harden, M.D., Director of the Pain Clinic at the Rehabilitation Institute of Chicago, supports this theory in his research.

- *Exercise enhances the production of T-cells.* It has been validated in research that, with exercise, the thymus gland releases a greater abundance of "killer T-cells" which boost the autoimmune system and are utilized to fight foreign cells and disease-threatening components in the body.

- *Exercise increases levels of serotonin and growth hormone.* Serotonin and the growth hormone are the exact pain reducing and muscle-repair hormones that people with fibromyalgia may lack. Exercise increases their production in the body.

- *Exercise increases the production and flow of synovial fluid into and out of the cartilage in the joints.* The consistent movement of synovial fluid into and out of the cartilage keep it healthy and well nourished. Healthy joints, of course, help to prevent or heal arthritis and are a great benefit to the fibromyalgia sufferer.

As stated earlier, exercise is one of the more beneficial components of the health and healing regimen for the fibromyalgia sufferer. The following list is a more complete list of the benefits of exercise. Exercise impacts the individual mentally, physically, and emotionally and will:

- Tone and strengthen every organ and system of your body.
- Relax tension and enhance deep sleep (level 4).
- Strengthen self control, increase mental efficiency and enhance the feeling of well being and emotional strength.
- Help ward off anxiety and depression.
- Promote relaxation.
- Lower blood fats (triglycerides) and increase good cholesterol (HDLs) thus helping to reduce your risk of coronary heart disease and stroke.
- Decrease insulin resistance, aid in the control of blood sugar levels, and aid in the treatment of diabetes.
- Improve elimination and relieve constipation.
- Protect you against osteoporosis and arthritis.
- Increase your strength and endurance for both work and play.
- Improve your body composition (lower body fat percent, increase muscle tissue).
- Lengthen your life expectancy.

THE VARIOUS AREAS OF PHYSICAL FITNESS

Understanding the right kinds of exercises for the best health recovery and maintenance program is not as simple as it might sound. Common questions are: How much exercise should I do? And when do I do it? Do I walk for heart health and do weight resistance exercises? Do I also have to do stretching and calisthenics? What do I really need do to do for my health and healing regimen?

Given that you already have pain in the muscles as a fibromyalgia sufferer, it would be very wise if you enlisted the service of your medical doctor who can help determine your general level of health and well-being. Your doctor, then, can recommend an exercise physiologist or a physical therapist who can help devise the proper exercise program for you based on your current condition with fibromyalgia and your doctor's specifications.

Let's look at areas of exercise and fitness that make up the complete program for both the average person seeking general fitness and the fibromyalgia patient. The three areas of exercise and fitness are cardiovascular fitness, muscular strength, and flexibility.

Cardiovascular Fitness

Cardiovascular fitness refers to your aerobic capacity—the ability of the heart and lungs to supply blood, oxygen, and nutrients for vigorous activity. Exercises that increase your cardiovascular fitness also strengthen the joints and improve bone health. Such results are encouraging because bone health helps to prevent osteoporosis, aids in weight control, prevents heart disease and lowers high blood pressure. Examples of cardiovascular fitness or aerobic type activities are brisk walking, biking, jogging, stair climbing, swimming, rowing, line dancing, and particular sports that involve continuous movement. The activity that affords the opportunity to get your heart rate in your target zone and keep it there for at least 20-25 minutes consistently is considered aerobic and beneficial to heart and lung health. (The formula for computing your personalized target heart rate will be provided in the walking section of this chapter.) The key here is finding the right activity and determining the level at which you can perform it. For example, depending upon the severity of your condition, you may need to begin with gentle walking on a treadmill or riding a stationary bike for only 5-10 minutes per session. You can start doing this 3-4 days per week and gradually increase over several weeks, working up to 25-30 minute sessions for 4-5 days per week.

Muscular Strength

Muscular strength is very important for preventing injuries while lifting, doing housework, participating in recreational activities, and exercising. Strength training is also called resistance training and involves repeatedly lifting a weight or moving against a "resistance." Lifting free weights like dumb bells or barbells, or using weight machines and resistance devices like elastic tubing are all examples of resistance exercises. You do not have to lift several hundred pounds to improve your strength. In fact, depending upon the severity of your condition, you may need to start with 5-10 pound weights or an equal resistance with an elastic tubing device, but the important thing is to get started at an appropriate, comfortable level and gradually progress. I would strongly recommend beginning your exercises with dumb bells (small light weights that can be held in one hand), weight machines, or elastic tubing resistance devices. These are much easier to work with and much safer than the larger, heavier free weights. Once you have significantly progressed and improved strength, then heavier and more difficult-to-handle free weights would be a more viable option.

Muscular Flexibility

Excellent muscular flexibility (stretchability) is very important in that relative inflexibility of muscles can cause excessive stress and force to be exerted on areas of the body opposite movement. This can very easily lead to injury and worsen the fibromyalgia condition. All types of movement, aerobic activities as well as strength development activities, can improve flexibility. However, some of the best flexibility exercises are yoga, various martial art forms, and all types of stretching. The more effective and efficient movements for flexibility are those utilizing stretch devices such as elastic tubing. The elastic tubing devices are especially effective because generally you can include both strength development and flexibility type movement.

ESTABLISHING YOUR EXERCISE PROGRAM

Muscle strengthening, cardiovascular, and stretching exercises can be performed safely and effectively by most fibromyalgia sufferers. Remember that common sense and moderation are always the rules when beginning an exercise program. Be certain that you contact your physician for a thorough examination and then consult with an exercise physiologist or physical therapist to assist you in tailoring an exercise program to your specific personal needs and limitations. Remember, if you have an acute flair up with your condition, your doctor or exercise physiologist might very well suggest that you do your exercises only on a stationary bike or participate in very low impact movement. You may even stop exercising for a short period of time until you can recover to the point that you can effectively begin again.

Beware of personal trainers who mean well but are not familiar with your condition and do not have formal training in designing programs for people with limitations. Also book-type programs for those who have no specific limitations should be avoided by those with fibromyalgia symptoms. A doctor, preferably a rheumatologist who has knowledge of fibromyalgia, should probably devise an exercise program for you following your physician's specifications.

Your health and healing exercise program should be designed so that you are gradually building up and doing more intense exercise for longer periods of time without straining or forcing the point of injury or causing undue pain. The program should include cardiovascular fitness, muscular strength, and muscular flexibility. The following are some guidelines to keep in mind as you proceed with your program:

121

- Utilize your natural biofeedback and listen to your body. Whenever you feel dizzy, become nauseated, experience an undue shortness of breath, or feel any pain in the body (especially the chest), then always stop your exercise immediately.
- Be sure that you avoid doing too much too soon so that you might avoid unnecessary injury. Remember there is a marked difference between pushing just a little more to improve and pushing yourself to the point of injury. Learn to establish the difference between the two.
- Learn to establish the difference between slight muscle soreness due to past workouts and aggravation of fibromyalgia pain.
- When beginning your exercise program, remember to go easy and to work at a comfort level, building gradually. Just remember that your body will adapt naturally. You will be amazed at how quickly and readily you will improve and be able to increase resistance and time.
- Always warm up very carefully, taking time to create blood flow and increased body heat in the muscle fiber. A proper warm up will insure a comfortable, enjoyable workout and help you to avoid unnecessary injury.
- A good rule of thumb is to always cool down gradually after exercising, not stop abruptly. Bring the heart rate and body temperature down gradually. A good way to cool down is to walk easily, stretch and shake out your arms and legs. The proper cool down will assist your body in dissipating lactic acid and will decrease the amount of muscle soreness. You will recover faster and be more refreshed for your exercise the next day.

EFFECTIVE EXERCISES

Cardiovascular activity, stretching, and weight resistance exercises using elastic tubing devices are the three most effective approaches to health improvement for most fibromyalgia sufferers. Weight training is the area in which we want to be most careful and begin more deliberately after improvement has been made in other areas of training. Below are some specific exercises listed with suggested guidelines for performing them safely.

Walking

Walking is one of the most complete, convenient, effective, easiest, and enjoyable ways to lose weight and restore and maintain total health. Not only does walking burn calories and fat, it also tones and strengthens muscles, boosts energy, and improves total health and well-being. Walking will improve muscle flexibility, help to eliminate early morning stiffness, alleviate muscle pain, and improve the overall muscle physiology for energy production—all major problems for the fibromyalgia victim.

There are some very important guidelines for you to follow to move you safely and efficiently toward your goal of health and healing. The most effective program combines the proper walking routine along with lifestyle changes like improved nutrition. The most effective way to burn the most calories and to lose weight healthfully and efficiently is to walk for a longer time and greater distances as opposed to walking faster and going shorter distances.

If time and distance are a problem in the beginning because of a lack of physical condition or obesity, begin with moderate times and distances. For instance, take ten, fifteen, or twenty minute walks initially. After a couple of weeks, do these short walks more than once a day until you can gradually increase your time to 30-45 minutes of continuous walking. For best results concerning weight loss and a healthy heart, you should be performing within your target heart rate zone which is somewhere between 50 percent and 70 percent of your maximum heart rate. To compute your target heart rate (THR), subtract your age from 220 and then subtract your resting heart rate (RHR); multiply by .5 and then add your resting heart rate back into the figure. The formula is as follows:

$$(220 - Age - RHR) \times .5 + RHR = THR$$

For instance, if you are 40 years of age, with a RHR of 65, your most efficient THR for weight loss is 123:

$$(220 - 40 - 65) \times .5 + 65 = 123$$

Walking and exercising within this heart rate range, you are giving yourself the best opportunity to walk extended periods without tiring and still efficiently lose weight and maintain a state of health.

Following this program consistently will assist you in logging 20 to 30 miles per week for a weekly energy expenditure of approximately 2000-3000 calories. If you will maintain this program consistently you can burn just under a pound of fat per week or 35 to 50 pounds a year. This can be computed very easily because approximately 3500 calories equals one pound.

The following are some tips to help ensure your success in your health restoring and walking program:

- *Energy, movement, and positive experiences:* Build your health-restoring program around exercise, energy, and positive thinking and it will help to enhance your success. Very often when we build restoring health and weight loss around food there is a tendency to think only about food. Walking for the restoring of health works not only physiologically but has a very strong impact psychologically. It begins to help restore self-esteem, it energizes, and raises our metabolism.

- *Think consistency and commitment:* If you made the commitment to do what is necessary on a daily basis with lifestyle changes to restore your health and vitality, then you are on your way to success. Writing your goals down will help to insure your success. (There are suggestions in Chapter 7 which will help you in the goal setting process.)

- *Walk six days a week:* You may read that three days a week is sufficient for good heart health. That may be true if you are only working toward maintaining good heart health, but remember you have made a commitment to restore your health. You have to be consistent with your lifestyle change in order to overcome the symptoms and conditions of fibromyalgia. If you set a goal to walk only three days a week it might become too easy to get away from your program by missing too many days. If you walk six out of seven days, on the other hand, it becomes part of your lifestyle. It becomes a habit and you will look forward to it. If you take a break and have one day per week off you'll be refreshed and then you will look forward to getting back with your program on the following day.

- *Exercise time and distance are the keys:* To burn more calories, to maintain a healthful weight, and to make the best progress toward restoring good health, the key is to walk consistently—go farther and not faster. Remember, depending on the severity of your condition, you may need to begin with several brief walks daily, even as short as 3 five-minute walks. Then you build up gradually so that your pace is comfortable and you do not lose the enjoyment of your walk as you gain benefits. The goal is to work up to the point that you are walking six days per week, at your median pace, 30-45 minutes per session burning maximum calories.

- *Don't get hung up on numbers:* Especially early in your exercise program, don't worry about inches and pounds. Simply focus on the enjoyment of your daily exercise regimen, begin to look forward to it, be consistent, stick with it. If you begin to focus on whether or not your are losing inches and pounds—especially early in a program—it can become very discouraging.

- *Warming up properly for walking:* Do not stretch. The proper way to warm up for walking is not stretching. You never stretch a cold muscle. The best way to warm up for walking is an easy, gentle walk in the beginning to increase blood flow and body temperature gradually. Then increase your walking pace gradually over a period of five or six minutes to a median pace at which you complete your entire walk. However, if you want to do a few gentle arm circles, body twists, and neck rolls to increase blood flow and raise the body temperature gradually and gently loosen muscles, ligaments, and tendons, feel free to do so for five or six minutes before beginning your gentle warm up walk. After you have completed your walk is the time to stretch for flexibility. (See the stretching section of this chapter.)

- *Shoes and clothes are important:* Wear loose fitting, comfortable clothes and light colors if the heat is severe. Walk in the early mornings and late evenings in extreme heat and high humidity. Shoes with good support are very important. Do not walk in old shoes that have been broken down or that have lost their flexibility. A good running shoe is ideal for the support for joints, ligaments, and tendons that you need for efficient walking.

- *Find flat solid surfaces to walk on:* One of the most pleasant places to walk is in your neighborhood where you have a flat, smooth, asphalt surface, trees and pleasant surroundings. Other good choices are malls, park trails, and jogging tracks.
- *Consult your physician:* As always, consult your physician before beginning any aspect of an exercise program. For instance, if you have any severe orthopedic problems, for instance the hip, knee, ankle, or another weight–bearing joint, then walking may not be the best exercise for you until those conditions are corrected. Two alternatives are water exercises and cycling.

In summary, a few of the very important benefits of walking are stronger, more flexible muscles, ligaments, and tendons, especially in the hips, lower limbs, and the lower back. The arms, shoulders, and upper back will benefit as well. This strength and flexibility improvement will enhance the physiology of the muscles, therefore reducing early morning stiffness and alleviating the pain suffered by fibromyalgia victims. Another benefit is that of improved self image and overall sense of well-being; improved cardiovascular fitness which improves stamina and endurance; decreased body fat and an increase in lean body tissue therefore improving metabolism; decreased heart disease and blood pressure risk; and reduction in stress and tension.

Aquatics

Swimming and water exercises are very advantageous to many chronic conditions and extremely popular with physical therapists, exercise physiologists, and physicians. Patients also enjoy the aquatic exercises for the benefits that they normally gain. However, I should initially point out that the fibromyalgia patient should proceed with extreme care as water resistance sometimes can be equal to heavy weight resistance similar to weight lifting exercises. Those with severe fibromyalgia conditions should proceed very cautiously and under the direction of a professional as vigorous activity or movement in water could worsen the fibromyalgia condition. The water therapy can be most beneficial, especially in heated pools. Also, all three types of exercise that are very important to the fibromyalgia sufferer—strength, flexibility, and aerobic—can be accomplished in the water. Just a last word of caution: remember all movement should be of a very low impact and therapeutic nature so as not to worsen the fibromyalgia condition.

Another advantage of aquatic activities and exercises is that they can be performed in shallow water or with flotation devices therefore not requiring that the participants be expert swimmers or even having the skill of swimming at all. The following is a list of the benefits derived from aquatic activities and exercises:

- The water provides stability and support which could be especially beneficial for a fibromyalgia sufferer who has an advanced or extreme condition.
- The therapeutic movements in the water will help to relieve stress and anxiety.
- The water exercises will promote relaxation in the muscles, therefore enhancing relief of pain.
- Stronger, more flexible muscles result from these activities.
- Healthier joints result, which aid both the fibromyalgia and the arthritic patient.
- When participating with a group, the social interaction

serves as a tremendous benefit in gaining emotional confidence and developing sociability.

- Improved confidence in the benefits of exercise and within self.
- Improved heart and lung capacity that enhances the health and healing of the entire body.
- More strength and flexibility at the muscle/connective tissue junction (where the seat of the fibromyalgia problem usually rests).
- An increase in the neurotransmitter serotonin and the growth hormone which will benefit the fibromyalgia condition tremendously.
- The stimulation of the production of T–cells enhancing a stronger immune system, thus creating more of an ability for the body to heal itself.

Understand that walking and stretching are the two most beneficial types of exercise, especially when strength exercises can be combined with the stretching. However, aquatic exercises are an excellent alternative and have the potential to deliver many benefits. If you have access to a pool, especially a heated pool, this can be an excellent alternative to intermingle with your walking and strength/flexibility exercises.

Cycling

Most people with fibromyalgia can usually walk for their exercise. However, if you have a very chronic and severe condition with a great deal of pain around the knees and in the hip joints, then cycling could be an excellent alternative because of the fact that your legs and hips are not responsible for supporting your weight. Cycling could be ideal for those who have lower back pain, and pain around the knee areas.

Cycling is also something that most everyone already knows how to do and there is the convenience of cycling either in the neighborhood or on a stationary bike right within the home.

Cycling is a tremendous heart and lung conditioner, and also strengthens the quadriceps (the thigh muscles) more than walking. These are the muscles that get you up stairs, assist you in lifting, and get you out of chairs. Cycling exercises will strengthen the muscles around the knee joints which will greatly benefit the pain areas around the knees. Take precaution and adhere to the following guidelines when cycling:

- Always warm up before every activity, even before cycling. Remember not to warm up by stretching. Do not stretch cold muscles. Warm up with gentle, low–impact body movements and/or easy walking or easy cycling without resistance on a stationary bike or on flat surfaces outside. This will gradually raise the body temperature and increase the blood flow slowly and systematically.
- If there is pain in the lower back and the knees, be sure not to add very much resistance at all in the beginning on a stationary bike and avoid hills and strenuous areas cycling outside. Do this until the legs, heart, and lungs become better conditioned and the pain feels much improved.
- The bicycle seat should be adjusted so that your leg very nearly straightens when the pedal is at the bottom of the rotation. This adjustment allows the greatest benefit for muscular development and for cardiovascular efficiency.
- Remember to build up your time and distance on a very gradual basis so as not to aggravate your fibromyalgia condition. You will know as you listen to your body when you can add speed, distance, or resistance. With all other aspects of your program, be certain to discuss this with your physician and proceed with his or her approval.

Stretching

Stretching is a vital part of any exercise program for those people with fibromyalgia. Sedentary living habits and increased inactivity are major contributors to the loss of flexibility. Fibromyalgia patients typically adopt more sedentary living habits and become more inactive than normal because of the pain and lack of energy that are usually associated with the condition. This inactivity causes muscles and connective tissue to lose their pliability and allows body fat to increase tremendously, and contributes to decreased flexibility (stretchability).

Most people tend to lack flexibility in the front of the hip or the back of the thigh, in the lower back and neck and shoulders. In order to increase overall body flexibility it is necessary to engage in basic flexibility exercises that will affect the large muscle groups of these areas. If stretching exercises are done properly there are tremendous benefits for the fibromyalgia patient. However, if done incorrectly they can do more harm than good and possibly even cause damage. The following are some guidelines to insure that you get maximum benefit from your flexibility program:

- *You must stretch on a daily basis.* In order to derive the most benefit from your flexibility program you must stretch on a daily basis. Make a commitment, do it consistently, and do it properly. Remember it takes time to make progress in flexibility, so be patient. Stretching is ideally done *after* your exercise session.
- *Never use stretching for your warm up.* Always warm up before beginning stretching. For instance, do some mild walking and mild calisthenics such as arm swings and body rotations to increase the blood flow and body temperature.

Ideally you would even break a sweat before beginning to stretch.

- *Get in the correct, comfortable position to begin your stretch.* Slowly and gently stretch the muscle or muscle group with which you are working. Avoid sudden, bouncing movements because this stimulates sensory receptors that shorten the muscle. This is counterproductive since the muscle you are attempting to stretch is now shorter. When the muscle is stretched slowly and gently, other sensory receptors are activated that override the initial stretch response and prevent muscle contraction. The muscle will relax and you can lengthen it without stress or strain of movement. In the beginning put a very gentle stretch on the muscle, making sure not to feel pain. After holding this gentle stretch position for 5-6 seconds, the muscle will seem to relax even more (this is called proprioceptive neuromuscular facilitation). Once you have stretched just a bit farther, gently and with ease, hold the complete stretch for about ten seconds, and then release it very gently and move slowly back to the original position making sure not to release rapidly.

- *Be careful to select very simple exercises to begin your stretching program for the major muscle groups.* (Some suggested exercises will be given at the end of this section.)

- *Remember to concentrate on relaxing the muscle being stretched, even as it is being stretched.* This will facilitate a more efficient, more comfortable, safer stretch.

- *Remember that stretching exercises are not meant to be competitive.* Avoid bouncing movements and strenuous stretches. When you feel pain that means you are overstretching and you are possibly inflicting damage to the muscle.

- *Remember that stretching progress will come very slowly.* Don't push or be over anxious.

STRETCHES FOR FIBROMYALGIA SUFFERERS

The muscle groups that fibromyalgia patients should concentrate on are the arms, shoulders, the neck and upper back, the lower back, the hips, the thighs, especially the hamstrings in the back of the thighs. The following are some stretches that will improve joint health and impact most of the major pain centers of fibromyalgia sufferers:

1. *The lower back and buttocks.* Lie on the floor, hands by your side, legs straight with feet together. When lying or sitting for stretches, it is best to perform them on carpet or an exercise pad. Slowly bring both knees toward the chest reaching with your hands just under the knees and pull them toward the chest, bringing both knees as near the chest as possible with a gentle stretch on the lower back and buttocks. Hold for 4-5 seconds, then try and stretch just a bit farther. Holding for about ten seconds in the stretch position relaxing the muscles that are being stretched as much as possible, then return slowly and gently back to the starting position. Take caution not to put weight on the back of your neck. Resting momentarily between each stretch, perform the movement three to four times. (NOTE: This stretch will affect the pain-sensitive points in the lower back and the center of the buttocks.)

2. *The hip extensor and lower back.* Lying on your back, extend arms straight out to the side with hands at the shoulder level. Raise the left leg up to a vertical position, keeping the leg straight, then twist the body to place your left foot over across the top of the body attempting to touch the right hand. If you cannot place the left foot into the right hand on the floor at first, then move the hand to meet the foot. Gently stretch for 4-5 seconds, and then as you relax the muscle you should be able to extend the stretch a slight bit farther for the ten-second count. Return to the starting position and repeat

on the opposite side. Bring the right foot up to a vertical position, twist body to the left and bring the right foot over and across the body into the left hand for the same count. Perform three stretches on either side while keeping trunk and arms on the mat.

3. *Hip flexors, hamstrings (the back of the thighs), and the lower back muscles.* Lying on your back with hands to side and legs fully extended with feet together. Bring left knee toward the chest while keeping the right leg extended, reaching with both hands underneath the knee and pull toward the chest for a gentle stretch position. Hold for the ten-second count and return slowly to the starting position. Repeat the movement with the opposite leg.

4. *The trunk rotators, neck, shoulder, and upper back muscles.* Sit on the carpet or the exercise pad, cross both legs with feet pulled as near the buttocks as possible, keeping body erect, twist to the right, moving both arms, head and neck with the trunk. With trunk, head, and neck rotated 90 degrees to the right, reach with right hand and grab upper left arm and pull arm and shoulder gently across the body increasing the stretch on the upper arm, shoulder, and upper back. Hold for the ten-second count and return slowly and easily to the starting position. Now repeat the same movement, twisting the trunk to the left, reaching with the left hand, grabbing the upper right arm and pulling it gently across the body for the ten-second count. (NOTE: This stretch is impacting the pain sensitive points in the upper back, over the shoulder blades, and the top of the shoulders and in the lower back.)

5. *The lower back and neck muscles.* Sitting with legs crossed and feet as near buttocks as possible, keep upper body straight and erect for the beginning position. Fold arms and bend gently forward attempting to touch the forehead where the legs are crossed in front of the body. Hold a gentle stretch for 8-10 seconds, then return easily and gently to the starting

position. Repeat the exercise three to four times. Be cautious not to bounce or strain. The movement should be steady and gentle.

6. *The hamstrings (the back of the thighs), the buttocks, and the lower back.* Sit on the floor with legs straight, body erect, and feet together. Keeping legs straight, slowly and gently reach forward with both arms putting a gentle stretch on the back of the thighs, the buttocks, and the lower back. Reach as far as possible with both hands together and hold for the ten-second count, then return slowly and gently to the starting position. Repeat the movement for three or four repetitions.

7. *The pectoral muscles (the chest), the upper back, and the neck muscles.* Starting position is standing directly behind a chair, reaching both hands to the top of the back of the chair and standing far enough away that the upper body is parallel to the floor. Keeping the body and arms straight, perform a gentle stretch from the lower back, bending the body toward the floor, moving the head down between the arms, holding on to the back of the chair, keeping the legs straight. While in the stretch position, move the head down farther, looking back toward the legs, with the head between the arms, placing a gentle stretch on the back of the neck muscles. Hold for the ten-second count and move easily and gently back to the starting position. Perform four repititions of the movement.

Strength Training

The best devices for strength training are resistance devices like elastic tubing with anchors that can be attached to doors or walls. Less desirable devices for the fibromyalgia patient would be free weights (dumb bells and barbells) or using weight machines. These can be used successfully, however, if you work with weights as light as 5-10 pounds and get professional help as to proper exercise regimens and techniques. Still, the most highly recommended weight resistance exercises are those that use elastic tubing. Exercises using elastic tubing are very light resistance, very flexible and very low impact. A tremendous advantage of the elastic tubing devices is that strength and flexibility movements are combined within the one device (Elrod, 1996). See Resource List in the back of this book for information on ordering my "Body Advantage" system, which includes an elastic tubing stretch device and video.

"STICKING WITH" YOUR PROGRAM

The key to sticking with your exercise program is to find exercises and a regimen or routine that you thoroughly enjoy. Develop a very positive attitude toward changing your lifestyle and toward exercise in general. Remember that it will be a key component in restoring your health and vitality. Experiment until you find the exercises and the situation that fits you. If you enjoy the water, then join a water exercise or swimming class. If you love the outdoors, then develop exercise regimens and routines outside. If you prefer to be inside, then develop a regimen and routine using exercise equipment, exercise cycles or join a dance class. Use the buddy system— exercise with a family member or a friend. Read or listen to music while you are exercising. Change your routine—change your walking route for variety. There are exercises, regimens, and routines that are perfect for you, so make them as pleasant and enjoyable as you possibly can and just do it.

- *Begin with a positive attitude.* The human mind is a fascinating organism. If you begin with negative thoughts and statements, soon you will succumb to the negativism. On the contrary, if you begin with positive attitudes and positive thinking you will purely and simply get positive results.
- *Begin properly.* Obtain professional help to be assured that you can begin your program safely and effectively. A large percentage of those who begin on their own do too much too soon and possibly can do more harm than good.
- *Organize your day and prioritize.* Many conclude "there are not enough hours in the day" or "I would love to, but I just simply do not have enough time." Simply set aside the time, making it a necessary and very important part of your lifestyle. Remember that it is one of the key components of your return to health and vitality.
- *Make it convenient and enjoyable.* Avoid cumbersome routines. Create workout areas right at home and mark off walking tracks and distances right in the neighborhood or nearby parks with pleasant, enjoyable surroundings.
- *Find your time of day.* Find the time of day that you function more efficiently and that works into your schedule most conveniently.
- *Vary your routine.* Do cross or seasonal training. This helps to prevent boredom and keeps you energized about your program. Cross training means that you are trying different activities like swimming, walking, or cycling. Change your routes or scenery while cycling or walking.
- *Back off on days that you're not quite feeling up to it.* Some days you just might not feel quite up to it so back off and reduce your workout time. Remember that "something is better than nothing." However, some days you might just want to reward yourself. Read a book, paint a picture, or go to a movie so that you continue to be motivated for your exercise routine.

- *Keep records and set goals.* A great incentive builder at times is to keep records of your program involvement. Maintain an interest in keeping up with what you do, how often, your progress, your personal comments, and results. Some enjoy taking body measurements, keeping up with blood pressure, change in resting heart rate, etc. Set some goals in these areas and keep up with those with which you have the greatest interest. (See daily log in Appendix A.)
- *Buy new shoes and clothes.* Maintain a reasonable budget, but reward yourself with walking and exercise shorts and clothes that are attractive, comfortable and motivating. Devices such as walkman radios and heart rate monitors can also be enjoyable and motivating.
- *Utilize the buddy system.* If you have a workout partner to join you and encourage you on a daily basis helps tremendously. Someone waiting for you will stimulate you to exercise on a more regular basis. Enjoying the company and conversation of a good friend or workout partner is something that keeps many people going with the program.

Exercise for Restored Health

It is advised that chronic pain sufferers should begin with gentle exercises such as easy stretches, slow low-impact walking, leisurely swimming, or light resistance exercises with elastic devices. By all means, get your physician's approval before starting any exercise program. Avoid specific exercises or activities that place abnormal stress on your muscles or joints and that cause more undue pain. However, the most critical thing to do is simply start exercising!

CHAPTER 7

Coping with Stress and Depression

Typically, anything that limits mobility, threatens disability, or produces pain can lead to increased stress and eventually to a state of depression. This in turn can result in fatigue, a lack of interest in family, friends, and even sexual activities, and many other problems. Depression is a very common side effect of fibromyalgia. It is a very natural response to be upset and stressed when pain forces one to give up favorite activities, makes routine chores difficult, and reminds one of its presence even when sitting or lying down. The risk of depression increases greatly as the threat of disability becomes apparent and as pain becomes more severe. When unpredictable pain flairups occur, the fibromyalgia victim tends to feel continuously threatened by the disease.

STRESS VS. DEPRESSION

Effective stress coping techniques can greatly assist the fibromyalgia patient in fighting depression. First, however, it is very important to understand the difference between stress and depression so that effective stress coping techniques can be employed. Recognize that stress is the response of the mind, body, and emotions to everyday happenings and the pressures of life. It is important to understand that stress is not the actual event, but it is our interpretation or our emotional reaction to the event. For example, a very active person might find a stress fracture injury very traumatic, while the next person may find it an opportunity to rest up and refresh the body while recovering. The situations are very similar, but it's how the individuals respond to the situation that determines the stress impact (O'Koon, 1996).

This explanation helps explain why some people become much more stressed by the pain, fatigue and other circumstances associated with fibromyalgia than do others. However, even among those that cope with fibromyalgia extremely well, it can still become a very stressful situation. The following are symptoms that will help you to know when you are overly stressed (Dexter & Brandt, 1994):

- irritability
- fatigue
- nervousness
- sweaty, clammy hand
- anxiety
- muscle tension
- nausea
- loss of appetite

Being overly stressed appears to eventually lead to depression if not managed properly. *Also, feeling overly stressed seems to signal certain neurotransmitters to release chemicals that tend to shock the body and weaken the immune system, thus mak-*

ing the fibromyalgia symptoms and circumstances worse and increasing the risk for other conditions and diseases.

In the 1920s, Dr. Hans Selye at the University of Prague did pioneering research demonstrating that emotions can cause illness (Simonton, Simonton, & Creighton, 1992). Dr. Selye's research has been supported in some more recent studies utilizing both laboratory animals and humans. Many of these studies have also begun to reveal the physiological process by which undue emotional responses or chronic stress can create a susceptibility to disease. The body is designed so that moments of stress, followed by a physical reaction or release of that stress will allow little harm; in fact, proper amounts of stress are healthy. However, when the physiological response to stress is not discharged, there is a negative cumulative effect on the body, referred to as chronic stress. Chronic stress is increasingly recognized as a highly significant factor influencing conditions such as fibromyalgia. Dr. Selye has also discovered that chronic stress suppresses the immune system, responsible for controlling cancerous cells and other dangerous microorganisms such as free radicals.

The correlation between health and stress is obvious—in fact, the majority of fibromyalgia victims I have worked with have experienced a traumatic experience which caused a long period of undue or chronic stress in their lives. Interestingly, current research appears to be establishing a link between traumatic experiences, chronic stress, and fibromyalgia. According to research and the observations of various physicians, it appears that disease is more likely to occur following highly stressful events than not. It has been documented by physicians that when their patients suffered major emotional upsets there is generally an increase, not only in diseases usually acknowledged to be susceptible to emotional influence, (i.e., high blood pressure, obesity, ulcers, headaches), but also in infectious diseases, backaches, and even accidents.

Dr. Thomas H. Holmes and his associates at the University of Washington School of Medicine undertook research to validate these observations. They set out to develop a process by which they could objectively measure the amount of stress or emotional upset in an individual's life. The doctors designed a scale that listed traumatic or highly stressful events along with numerical values. The scale they developed follows: (Simonton, Simonton, & Creighton, 1992).

SOCIAL READJUSTMENT RATING SCALE

EVENT	VALUE
Death of a spouse	100
Divorce	73
Marital separation	65
Jail term	63
Death of a close family member	63
Personal injury or illness	53
marriage	50
Fired from work	47
Marital reconciliation	45
Retirement	45
Change in family member's health	44
Pregnancy	40
Sex difficulties	39
Addition to family	39
Business readjustment	39
Change in financial status	38
Death of close friend	37
Change to different line of work	36
Change in # of marital arguments	36
Mortgage or loan over $10,000	31
Foreclosure of mortgage or loan	30
Change in work responsibilities	29
Son or daughter leaving home	29
Trouble with in-laws	29
Outstanding personal achievement	28
Spouse begins or stops work	26

Starting or finishing school	26
Change in living conditions	25
Revision of personal habits	24
Trouble with boss	23
Change in work hours, conditions	20
Change in residence	20
Change in schools	20
Change in recreational habits	19
Change in church activities	19
Change in social activities	18
Mortgage or loan under $10,000	17
Change in sleeping habits	16
Change in number of family gatherings	15
Change in eating habits	15
Vacation	13
Christmas season	12
Minor violation of law	11

This scale includes highly stressful events as well as what would be perceived as happy events, such as marriage and promotions. The point is that even though they are positive experiences, they still demand a great deal of thought and adjustment and may cause unresolved emotional conflict within an individual. The ability to adapt to change is required in every stressful situation, whether it be positive or negative.

Not surprisingly, fibromyalgia is generally viewed as a negative stressor, as is most anything that threatens disability, produces pain, and limits one's ability to function normally. Depression is a common side effect. Many researchers, in fact, believe that when one is threatened with disability or loss of normal function, this is much more likely to induce depression than is the pain from the condition itself (Simonton & Simonton 1975).

The condition depression generally includes a wide variety of emotional disorders ranging from mild to severe. There are three basic levels of severity. First, people become depressed on a one-time only basis. The depression can last for a day, a few days, or several weeks and then never return. Second, recurrent depressive disorders can appear and disappear periodically, leaving one feeling very good and normal between the episodes of depression. Finally, chronic depressive disorders can last for several years, maybe even for half a lifetime. Very often the symptoms are more severe in the first two to four years.

What doctors call subclinical depression is not serious enough to lead to diagnosis or treatment. Clinical depression, however, means that your symptoms are serious enough to warrant medical attention and treatment. Only your physician or psychologist should make that determination. Remember, however, if the number of subclinical symptoms continues to increase, or if they seem to become more severe, then treatment could be warranted in this case as well (O'Koon, 1996).

RECOGNIZING THE SYMPTOMS OF DEPRESSION

If the symptoms of depression, which many of us experience quite often, do not seem to go away and seem to worsen, then you could possibly truly have the condition of depression. The following is a list of the symptoms of depression to look for. If one or more of these symptoms seem to hang on for an extended period of time then you should contact your physician right away (Fries, 1995):

- loss of interest in the things you normally enjoy
- lack of interest in sex

- irritability or blue moods
- restlessness or a slowed-down feeling
- feelings of worthlessness or guilt
- appetite changes leading to weight gain or loss
- suicidal thoughts or thoughts of dying
- problems with concentration, thinking, or memory
- difficuty making decisions
- lack of sleep, or sleeping too much
- constant lack of energy
- headaches not caused by any other disease or condition
- other aches and pains not caused by any other condition
- digestive problems unrelated to any other condition
- feelings of hopelessness
- anxiety
- low self-esteem
- nightmares, especially with themes of loss, pain, or death
- preoccupation with failure, illness, etc.
- fear of being alone

Who Is At High Risk for Depression?

Physicians and psychologists have identified specific risk factors that increase the odds of depression (O'Koon 1996). These apply to the general population and not just fibromyalgia and osteoarthritis sufferers. The risk is increased for depression if you:

- are a woman
- have had a prior depressive episode
- had your first depressive episode before you were age forty
- have a medical condition
- have just given birth
- have very little or no social support

- have undergone a stressful life event (positive or negative)
- abuse alcohol or drugs
- have a family history of depressive disorders
- received only partial relief from an earlier episode of depression
- have made prior suicide attempts

The above list of risk factors only helps identify those who are more susceptible to depression. They do not mean that if you have some of those risk factors in your life that you are absolutely doomed to depression. It also does not mean that you are guaranteed a depression-free life if the list does not describe you. If you feel that you could possibly be depressed, get medical help immediately and possibly a referral to a therapist. Since certain drugs can help cause depression, inform your physician of the medications that you are currently or have recently been taking.

Stress Analysis

The following stress analysis questionnaire was specifically designed to assist you with your health status evaluation. Please be precise and objective with your answers. They should describe your exact present condition and not as you would prefer to be. Analyze your answers related to your total health state and you may, in fact, discover some stressful areas of which you were unaware, thus assisting you in coping more effectively and enhancing the potential of improving your personal health (Elrod, 1996).

Stress Risk Factors:
- _ Headaches
- _ Neck Pain
- _ Shoulder Pain
- _ Auto Accident
- _ Work Injury
- _ Backaches
- _ Other

Complete the following questions. If the answer is "maybe," check yes.

Yes No

1. Are you generally dissatisfied with your job, occupation, or relations with the opposite sex?
2. Do you have trouble relaxing or falling asleep?
3. Do you have trouble concentrating or remembering things?
4. Do you feel fatigued late in the day?
5. Do you have headaches, neck or back pain more than two times monthly?
6. Do you take pain relievers, antacids, tranquilizers, sinus or any other relief oriented medicine more than two times monthly?
7. Do you have insomnia or don't sleep enough?
8. Do you depend on sugar of caffeine stimulants?
9. Do you lose your temper or become angry easily?
10. Have you suffered a significant loss in the last year: job, money, divorce, death of loved one?
11. Do you eat red meat daily?
12. Is you weight abnormal?
13. Are you moody?
14. Are you hyper-active?
15. Do your hands or feet ever tingle, ache, burn ?
16. Do you have high blood pressure, heart disease, ulcers, colitis, or other stress related diseases?
17. Is there conflict, upset, or disappointment in a close personal relationship?
18. Does eating lack enjoyment?
19. Do you crave sugar?

General Stress

1. Do you take laxatives?
2. Would you call yourself a worrier?
3. Do you crave sweets?
4. Do you get tired after you eat sweets?
5. Do you find it difficult to work under pressure?
6. Do you develop bruises for no reason?
7. Do you have brown spots on your skin?

147

_ _ 8. Do cuts or scrapes heal slowly?
_ _ 9. Does your skin itch?
_ _ 10. Is your sex drive low?
_ _ 11. Do you suffer from skin rashes?
_ _ 12. Do you smoke?
_ _ 13. Do you suffer from acne?
_ _ 14. Do you or have you had bladder/kidney infections?

Immune Stress

_ _ 1. Do you get ear infections often?
_ _ 2. Do you suffer with sinus problems?
_ _ 3. Do you have chronic cough?
_ _ 4. Do you get chest colds often?
_ _ 5. Do you get sore throats often?
_ _ 6. Do you catch colds easily?
_ _ 7. Do you sigh or yawn often?
_ _ 8. Are you chronically tired?
_ _ 9. Do you have frequent allergies?
_ _ 10. Do you have indigestion or cold sores frequently?

Digestive Stress

_ _ 1. Do you have a poor appetite?
_ _ 2. Do you experience digestive problems when eating fatty or greasy foods?
_ _ 3. Do you suffer from nausea?
_ _ 4. Does food feel like it lays on your stomach?
_ _ 5. Do you have bad breath?
_ _ 6. Do you have loose bowel movements?
_ _ 7. Are you troubled by heartburn?
_ _ 8. Are you troubled by belching or gas?
_ _ 9. Do you suffer from constipation?
_ _ 10. Have you lost your taste for food?

Circulatory Stress

_ _ 1. Do you ever get light-headed or dizzy?
_ _ 2. Do you get pain or tightness in your chest?
_ _ 3. Do you have low blood pressure?
_ _ 4. Do you have high blood pressure?
_ _ 5. Do you get short of breath easily?
_ _ 6. Do you take prescription heart medication?

_ _ 7. Does your heart beat fast for no reason?
_ _ 8. Are your ankles swollen in the morning?
_ _ 9. Do you have varicose veins?
_ _ 10. Do you get dizzy when changing position?

Endocrine Stress

_ _ 1. Do you get depressed easily?
_ _ 2. Do you find it difficult to relax?
_ _ 3. Do you lose your temper easily?
_ _ 4. Do you cry easily?
_ _ 5. Do you find it hard to concentrate?
_ _ 6. Are you in menopause?
_ _ 7. Do you have pain with your cycle?
_ _ 8. Do you have "abnormal" menstrual flow?
_ _ 9. Do you have an "irregular" menstrual cycle?
_ _ 10. Do you get tired before you eat?
_ _ 11. Do you have lumps in your breasts?
_ _ 12. Do you suffer from insomnia?
_ _ 13. Do you gain weight easily?
_ _ 14. Do you find it difficult to gain weight?
_ _ 15. Do you suffer from headaches?

If you answered yes to three or more of the questions in any one category, lifestyle changes within that area are probably in order for improvement of your general well-being. The answers you provide in this analysis are important in understanding related health matters.

Program for Personal Stress Management

Stress is a physiological and emotional response from within, not just an event that has occurred. This indicates with good stress management techniques and proper programming of the subconscious mind, you can control stress. Stress is a physical or psychological threat, even if imaginary; however, real or imaginary, the body responds the same.

Sources of and Suggestions for Dealing with Stress

Recognizing situations that are personally stressful is an important first step. How you choose to deal with each is even more important. The following are areas of life that can be stress producing:

1. *Financial affairs.* Avoid debt, manage finances, use discipline within a realistic budget.
2. *Family life.* Work at healthy relationships, communication skills, and the art of giving.
3. *Personal and Social Life.* Develop a support system through friends and hobbies. Do not harbor resentment, be forgiving, and work at boosting your self-esteem.
4. *Physical problems.* Have medical check-ups regularly. If you are experiencing constant fatigue, check your rest habits, improve your nutrition, and take supplements in the form of vitamins, minerals, and herbs. Exercise regularly, a minimum of 4 or 5 times per week. Seek professional advice in all the above areas.
5. *Work life.* If you are unhappy with your work, investigate continuing education and job training opportunities to improve where you are. If you strongly feel you are misplaced, then courageously seek your purpose and pursue your new mission with a passion. Consider your work as a joy and pleasure.
6. *Change.* Change is inevitable, therefore develop a positive

attitude toward change. Remember that change can be healthy. Take care to make changes slowly and not too many at once, so as to ensure success.

7. *Time pressures.* Much of our stress is caused by mismanagement of time, procrastination, and deadlines.

Since stress can lead directly to depression, we need to focus on how to overcome stress. One of the keys to successful stress coping is to develop the positive habit pattern of awakening each day with a thankful heart and an optimistic attitude. As you first begin to gain consciousness in the early morning the functioning of the subconscious mind is at the alpha level, 10-12 brain wave lengths per second. The subconscious mind at the alpha level is more sensitive and receptive to thoughts, emotions, and aspirations than at any other time. Therefore, it is at this part of the day that you want to *visualize* yourself pain free, happy, optimistic, productive, and successful. These thoughts and aspirations will go with you throughout the day. Also remember that your very thoughts and emotions are triggering the release of endorphins and catecholamines, the healing and uplifting hormones within your immune system. The wonderful news is that by focusing on all that is hopeful, joyful, pleasant, loving, and optimistic, you can take the edge off stress and continuously improve the condition and state of fibromyalgia as you consistently move back toward a healthy existence. The list below contains some other guidelines for a healthful stress coping program:

- Boost your nutrition by eating more frequently, 4-5 times per day, eat with balance choosing an abundance of complex carbohydrates and high fiber foods such as whole grains, whole grain breads and cereals, rice, pasta, beans, peas, and potatoes, along with plenty of fresh fruits and vegetables with only 20 percent of your total volume being fat. Avoid sugar, caffeine, and stay away from sugar-laden false foods, fat, and desserts.

- Vitamin and mineral supplements of any antioxidant combination will boost the immune system and enhance the cellular cleansing process by maintaining and invigorating cellular energy, cardiovascular awareness, and youthful vitality.

- Get regular exercise. Exercise aerobically by cycling, walking, or swimming a minimum of four to five times per week. Also, include stretching and muscle toning exercises two to three days per week. Joint stretching and muscle toning exercises will be very beneficial and remember that exercising regularly will increase the potential for the fibromyalgia victim to move into deep sleep while resting.

- Balance rest and relaxation with your exercise and activity. Be sure to get adequate amounts of sleep, focus on the positive, work at sleeping peacefully by going through your relaxation exercises while visualizing your goals. Remember that rest and relaxation will help to reduce muscle tension which will help in reducing pain.

- It is important to avoid prescription tranquilizers and sleeping medications of the benzodiazeprene group. While these may help you get to sleep, they will suppress deep sleep and therefore often make fibromyalgia symptoms worse the next day. Alcohol or narcotic pain medications taken in the evenings have the same effect on deep sleep and also should be avoided.

- Practice good stress management techniques. Don't over extend yourself and always plan ahead for difficult tasks and remember to ask for help whenever needed. Limit your responsibilities and activities to easily manageable levels.

- Be especially moderate with caffeine and alcoholic beverages and do not use drugs unless necessitated and prescribed by your doctor.

- Ingest a reasonable number of calories to enhance your weight loss and/or weight maintenance program.

STRESS REDUCING TECHNIQUES

The art of relaxation is most important in stress management and can be a structured or an informal technique. The following are some proven stress reducing activities: gentle stretching, a warm bath, breathing and muscle relaxation techniques, a brief nap, a walk in the woods, ocean sounds, nature sounds, and relaxing music, doing a favor for a friend, using humor frequently, meditation, prayer, mental relaxation, and using a foot massager.

NUTRITION GUIDELINES

- Avoid skipping meals, especially breakfast
- Limit the intake of sugar and highly refined foods
- Limit fat intake to 20 percent of the total calories
- Increase fiber in the form of fruits, vegetables, breads, cereals, legumes (do this gradually so as to avoid bloating)
- Maintain appropriate weight with a balance of 70 percent carbohydrates, 20 percent fats, and 10 percent protein on a daily basis
- Modify intake of red meat, caffeine, alcohol.
- Eliminate NutraSweet (use honey or fructose).
- Take supplements, including antioxidants. The minimum suggested amounts daily are 1,000 mg of vitamin C, 800 IU of vitamin E, 25,000 IU of beta carotene, 50 mg of coenzyme Q-10, and 100 mg per fifty pounds of body weight of pycnogenol (proanthocyanidins).
- Drink 72 ounces of purified (not tap) water daily . If you have no choice but to take tap water, refrigerate it to allow the chlorine and other impurities to dissipate. Water in tea and other drinks does not count toward the above.

REST, WORRY AND STRESS

Rest is as vital as exercise and nutrition for general health and combating stress. Research indicates that adults require between six and eight hours of sleep. You should determine whether you require six, seven, or eight hours through experimentation and monitoring your sleep over a prolonged period. When you have adequate sleep and the body is rested, you will wake up naturally without an alarm. Try the following for improved rest:

- Exercise regularly (not too close to bedtime).
- Avoid eating and ingesting stimulants after 6:00 p.m.
- Bedroom should be quiet and dark.
- Establish pre-sleep routine (i.e., reading, meditating, praying, etc.).
- Refrain from taking sleeping pills (take vitamins and nutrients instead).
- Organize concerns and develop action plans with objectivity rather than worry.
- Always plan your day in the afternoon or evening of the day before—not the morning of that day.

Fibromyalgia can produce a host of psychological changes due to anxiety, frustration, pain, depression, and stress. The reversing fibromyalgia regimen and approach will assist you in healthfully managing stress and avoiding depression in several ways. By utilizing your total fibromyalgia treatment program of nutrition, exercise, and suggested supplements, along with the stress coping methods and techniques in this chapter, you should be able to combat stress and overcome and avoid depression.

CHAPTER 8

Natural Supplements and Herbal Remedies

More and more physicians are becoming interested in alternative and natural treatments that utilize the products of Mother Nature. This is primarily a result of the positive data underscoring their effectiveness in helping people regain and maintain their health and vitality. At the same time, the conventional physician may not be that knowledgeable about natural treatments because of limited time. The average physician is hard pressed just to keep up on all the new drugs, let alone study all the breakthroughs on herbs, vitamins, minerals, supplements and nutritional treatments.

People with fibromyalgia and other chronic conditions should use caution when self-treating without the guidance of a physician or health professional who is well trained in nutrition. There are so many products and so much information available that it is easy to be confused about what to use and how to use it. However, with proper guidance, you can be successful in returning to vibrant health and an active lifestyle. The following is a more complete list and description of the minerals, vitamins, herbs, and supplements that may be helpful for fibromyalgia and other systemic conditions.

MINERALS ARE CRUCIAL

Much research has been done regarding the importance of minerals in the body and their function in healthy development. Minerals are absolutely the most important of all the body's nutrients. Even though the body needs only small amounts of many minerals, they need to be supplied on a daily basis to maintain and regulate necessary body functions. It is necessary to supplement the diet with minerals and other nutrients. Minerals are key because vitamins, amino acids, enzymes, fats, and carbohydrates all require minerals for their activity. Without minerals, they cannot be absorbed and utilized.

Minerals are also necessary for normalizing the heartbeat, improving the brain and mental abilities, stabilizing the nervous system, increasing energy and fighting fatigue, balancing electrolyte levels, and assisting the metabolic process. There are 84 known minerals, 17 of those being essential. If there is a shortage of one or more, the balance of the body's systems can be thrown off. One of the vital functions of minerals is that they assist in the regulation of the delicate balance of body fluids. They are vitally important in the process of osmosis which includes emptying the body of waste and bringing oxygen and nutrients to the cells. Minerals are purely and simply essential for all mental and physical functions.

More and more people are suffering from mineral deficiencies as minerals continue to disappear from our soils and food supply. This appears to be one of the major problems of the fibromyalgia sufferer. After long periods of undue stress and emotional disruption there is almost always a deficiency of some of the minerals, especially magnesium.

Minerals are disappearing from our food supply faster than updated charts can be published. Tables showing the nutrient content of foods can no longer be relied upon because of this fact. There is also a great variation of mineral content of foods because they are being grown under different conditions and in different locations. If minerals are scarce in plants, they are also scarce in human bodies. Mineral deficient plants also tend to be deficient in vitamins and in protein. It's a known fact that the amino acid component of protein is what forms neurotransmitters and neurotransmitters are vital to mental functioning. When there is a deficiency of minerals, the result is a nutritional imbalance that can lead to a disruption of sleep patterns, concentration, and the ability to interact normally (Weintraub, 1997). Growing evidence supports the fact that stress and anxiety over long periods of time result in mineral imbalances and this appears to be one of the primary factors that promotes the onset of fibromyalgia.

Research is being done on the importance of various minerals and it now appears that iron and iodine are very important as trace minerals. Chromium, zinc, manganese, magnesium, and copper also appear to be essential to good health. The following is a list of the important minerals and their nutritional value for the fibromyalgia sufferer and others with chronic conditions (Tenney, 1995).

MAGNESIUM

Magnesium is a major regulator of cellular activity, including the maintenance of DNA and RNA, and it is considered an anti-stress mineral. For this reason magnesium has a calming effect and is effective when taken before bedtime. Magnesium is an essential part of the enzyme system but is poorly assimilated by the body, so it should be taken daily by the fibromyalgia sufferer. A chocolate craving is sometimes indicative of a magnesium deficiency and deficiencies are very common in times of stress, malabsorption, diarrhea, diabetes, and kidney disease. This important mineral assists in the absorption of potassium, calcium, phosphorus, sodium, B-complex vitamins, as well as vitamins C and E. Some of the other symptoms of deficiency are weakness, depression, apprehension, irritability in the nerves and muscles, nausea, vomiting, sensitivity to noise, and muscle cramps and insomnia.

CALCIUM

Calcium is critically essential because it is the most abundant mineral in the body. Most of the calcium in the body is located in the bones and the teeth. It is necessary for the transmission of nerve signals and important for the smooth functioning of the heart muscles and muscular movements of the intestines. It is very important for good health, especially if one has a poor diet, suffers from malabsorption, or gets little sunshine. Calcium should be balanced with magnesium for proper nerve function and for a healthy body. Calcium, magnesium, and zinc all have a calming effect in the body and are very effective if taken before bedtime to help relax muscles and promote sleep. Vitamins A, C, D and phosphorus are also essential for the efficient functioning of calcium. Some of the symptoms of a calcium deficiency are tingling of the lips, fingers and feet, leg numbness, muscle cramps, and sensitivity to noise. (NOTE: Do not take antacids to make up for calcium deficiency.)

POTASSIUM

Potassium is responsible for normal heart and muscle function, normal transmission of nerve impulses, and normal growth. It works with sodium to regulate the flow of nutrients in and out of the cells and also helps to stimulate the kidneys, keep the adrenals healthy, and is involved in the maintenance of heart rhythm. Potassium is vital in stimulating nerve impulses which cause muscle contraction. The symptoms of a potassium deficiency include muscle twitches, weakness and soreness, erratic and/or rapid heartbeats, fatigue, glucose intolerance, nervousness, high cholesterol, and insomnia.

CHROMIUM

Chromium is essential for the synthesis of fatty acids and the metabolism of blood sugars for energy. It is also known for increasing the efficiency of insulin in carbohydrate metabolism. Symptoms of a deficiency include weight loss, glucose intolerance, and psychological confusion.

SELENIUM

Selenium is considered an aid to other nutrients, especially vitamin E. It is considered a very powerful antioxidant and needed for immune function, cell membrane integrity, and for DNA metabolism. Selenium is another mineral considered very important for systemic conditions as it protects the body from the toxicity of drugs and heavy metals such as aluminum, cadmium, and mercury.

ZINC

Zinc is a vital component of enzymes in the brain that repair cells. It is very important for hearing, vision, taste, and helps to form skin, hair, and nails. Zinc also assists with the absorption of vitamins in the body and is essential for the many enzymes involved in digestion and metabolism. Vitamin A must be present for zinc to be properly absorbed by the body. Symptoms of a deficiency include depression, distorted taste sensation, diarrhea, brittle nails and hair, hair loss, fatigue, and memory loss.

MANGANESE

Manganese is found in many enzymes in the body and assists in the utilization of glucose. It also aids in reproduction and normal functioning of the central nervous system. Manganese is also vital for proper brain function, muscles, nerves and is very important for energy production. Some of the symptoms of a deficiency are nausea, dizziness, muscle coordination problems, strained knees, loss of hearing, slow growth of hair and nails, and low cholesterol.

PHOSPHORUS

Phosphorus and calcium work together and are found mainly in the bones and teeth. Phosphorus levels can be decreased by drinking too much soda pop, a lack of vitamin D, and stress. Phosphorus is essential for fibromyalgia sufferers because it helps to produce energy as it aids in the oxidation of carbohydrates. Some of the symptoms of a phosphorus deficiency are a loss of appetite, irregular breathing, nervous disorders, and insomnia.

IODINE

The body requires very little of the trace mineral iodine, but it is essential for the thyroid hormone thyroxine. When supported by iodine, the thyroid gland helps to facilitate energy production. A malfunctioning thyroid can, of course, cause additional symptoms of fatigue and lethargy. Other symptoms of iodine deficiency are swollen fingers and toes, dry hair, cold hands and feet, and irritability.

IRON

Iron is a mineral that everyone is very familiar with yet many people suffer a deficiency in their nutritional programs. Iron is not easily absorbed by the body and requires an adequate amount of hydrochloric acid for proper assimilation. Vitamins C and E are also necessary if iron is to be utilized efficiently. Iron is known as the anti-anemia mineral because of its assistance in the oxygenation of cells and combining with protein to form hemoglobin.

VANADIUM

There is not a great deal of information available on vanadium, yet much evidence points to the fact that this trace mineral probably assists in preventing heart disease. Vanadium is a cofactor to insulin and, along with chromium, is very efficient in breaking down fats and sugars helping to keep coronary arteries clear. This mineral is vital in the creation of energy.

THE NATURE OF VITAMINS

A significant number of people with fibromyalgia and other systemic conditions are suffering from vitamin deficiencies. Vitamins are complex organic substances necessary for life and good health. Vitamins are constantly used in the body and must be replaced daily. They must be obtained from the food we eat, herbs, and supplements. Vitamins are necessary for the body to utilize other nutrients. They contribute to breaking down fats, carbohydrates, and protein into usable forms.

There are two types of vitamins, fat soluble and water soluble. Water soluble means they combine with water in the body to function and then are excreted in the urine. Most vitamins fall into the water soluble category. They only remain in the system for two to three hours so must be taken regularly whether in food or as a nutritional supplement. The fat-soluble vitamins are A, D, K, and E. They combine with the fats to be absorbed in the body and remain in the body for a much longer period of time. Vitamins should normally be taken before meals in order for proper absorption to take place. The following information will be beneficial to the person with fibromyalgia and those with other systemic conditions:

VITAMIN A

Remember that vitamin A is one of the fat-soluble vitamins and can be toxic within the body if taken in large quantities. However, beta carotene is nontoxic and is converted to vitamin A in the body on an as-needed basis. This is why one can take up to 25,000 I.U. of beta carotene on a daily basis and not build up a toxic effect. This vitamin helps maintain and repair muscle tissue, treats skin problems, fights infection, and aids in the growth and maintenance of healthy bones, skin, teeth, and gums. Some good sources of vitamin A are yellow and green vegetables, eggs, milk, liver, fish liver oils, carrots, apricots, and sweet potatoes. Some symptoms of a vitamin A deficiency include dry hair, itchy and burning eyes, sinus trouble, and fatigue.

VITAMIN C (ASCORBIC ACID)

Vitamin C is a water-soluble vitamin that is essential to the body. It helps prevent infection by increasing the activity of white blood cells and assists in destroying viruses and bacteria. It also performs as a powerful antioxidant and is considered an anti-stress vitamin. Vitamin C is essential for healing and the synthesis of neurotransmitters in the brain and, when combined with bioflavonoids, also assists with adrenal and immune functions. It helps in the formation of collagen which is essential for good skin, bones, teeth, and growth in children.

The following conditions usually call for an increase in vitamin C: infections, fevers, injuries, excessive physical activity, anemia, and cortisone use. Excellent sources of vitamin C include citrus fruits, cantaloupe, vegetables, broccoli, cauliflower, and red and green peppers. Some herbs that are good vitamin C sources are hawthorne berries, passionflower, olive oil, ginseng, and horsetail.

VITAMIN E (TOCOPHEROL)

One of the tremendous values of vitamin E for fibromyalgia sufferers is that it assists them in calming down and relaxing. Selenium increases the effectiveness of vitamin E and it is activated by vitamin A. It helps control the unsaturated fats in the body and is thought to reduce cholesterol, helps to normalize brain function, and protects glands during stress. Vitamin E is also considered one of the powerful antioxidants and is needed for cholesterol metabolism, blood clotting, lung metabolism, muscle and nerve maintenance, and body cleansing. Some good sources of vitamin E are peanuts, vegetable oils, lettuce, wheat germs, whole grains, spinach, corn, and egg yolks. The herb kelp is plentiful in vitamin E.

B-COMPLEX VITAMINS

Fibromyalgia patients need more B vitamins since they are under a great deal of stress and B vitamins assist in the calming process and good mental health. They are also vital in the production of serotonin, a chemical in the body that influences calming behavior. When B vitamins are deficient due to inadequate nutrition or increased demand it can significantly contribute to the lack of an ability to handle stress. B-complex vitamins work together to calm the nervous system and support correct brain function as well as to improve concentration and memory. Much care should be taken when taking the B vitamins as too much vitamin B6 is capable of causing a folic acid deficiency.

VITAMIN B1 (THIAMINE)

Vitamin B1 is necessary for digestion, blood cell metabolism, muscle metabolism, pain inhibition, and energy. B1 is a water soluble vitamin and needed in only small amounts on a daily basis. Some good sources of B1 are rice bran, wheat germ, oatmeal, whole wheat, sunflower seeds, brewer's yeast, and peanuts. Herbs that contain vitamin B1 are gotu kola, kelp, peppermint, slippery elm, and ginseng.

VITAMIN B2 (RIBOFLAVIN)

Vitamin B2 is necessary for antibody formation, red blood cell formation, cell respiration, fat and carbohydrate metabolism. B2 is also water soluble and must be replaced on a daily basis. It is also essential for proper enzyme formation, normal growth, and tissue formation. Some good sources of vitamin B2 are wild rice, liver, fish, white beans, sesame seeds, wheat germ, and red peppers. A few of the herbs containing B2 are gotu kola, kelp, peppermint, and ginseng.

VITAMIN B3 (NIACINAMIDE)

Vitamin B3 assists the body in producing insulin, female and male hormones, and thyroxine. B3 is also needed for circulation, acid production, and histamine activation. Some good sources of vitamin B3 are white meat, avocados, whole wheat, prunes, liver, and fish. Symptoms of a B3 deficiency are hypoglycemia, memory loss, irritability, confusion, diarrhea, ringing in the ears, depression, and insomnia.

VITAMIN B6 (PYRIDOXINE)

Vitamin B6 is helpful in converting fats and proteins into energy and with the production of red blood cells. It is also essential for proper chemical balance in the body. B6 is especially helpful to the fibromyalgia sufferer who is experiencing excessive stress. Symptoms of a B6 deficiency include irritability, nervousness, depression, muscle weakness, pain, headaches, PMS, and stiff joints.

VITAMIN B12 (COBALAMIN)

Vitamin B12 is essential for iron absorption; fat, protein, and carbohydrate metabolism; blood cell formulation; and long life of cells. A strict vegetarian will need to supplement with vitamin B12. Some symptoms of a B12 deficiency include headaches, memory loss, dizziness, paranoia, muscle weakness, fatigue, and depression.

BIOTIN

Biotin is especially needed if you are under excessive stress, experiencing malabsorption, or have a poor nutrition program. Biotin aids in protein, fat, and carbohydrate metabolism, fatty acid production, and cell growth. Some of the symptoms of a biotin deficiency are muscle pain, nausea, anemia, fatigue, high cholesterol, and depression.

PANTOTHENIC ACID

Pantothenic acid is needed for the normal functioning of muscle tissue and protects membranes from infection. It is also essential for energy conversion, blood stimulation, and detoxification. Individuals under excessive stress and with poor diets need pantothenic acid to assist in normal body functioning. Symptoms of a deficiency include digestive problems, muscle pain, fatigue, depression, irritability, and insomnia. Pantothenic acid is vital for the fibromyalgia sufferer due to the above facts.

PARA AMINOBENZOIC ACID (PABA)

PABA assists in facilitating protein metabolism, promoting growth, and blood cell formation. Some of the symptoms of a PABA deficiency are depression, fatigue, irritability, nervousness, constipation, and, in the long run, arthritis.

VITAMIN P (BIOFLAVONOIDS)

Bioflavonoids work together with vitamin C to strengthen connective tissue and capillaries. Bioflavonoids are also essential to assist the body in utilizing most of the other nutrients. Good sources of bioflavonoids are spinach, cherries, rosehips, citrus fruits, apricots, blackberries, and grapes. Herbs that contain bioflavonoids are paprika and rosehips.

HERBAL SUPPLEMENTS

Mother Nature provides herbs that have been used by mankind as healing agents since the dawn of history. In ancient times people were not aware that all the chemical elements contained in the leaves, root, bark, fruits, and flowers of herbs are the same chemicals that make up the human body. Modern technology has substantiated the use of herbal medicines and has proven why they have been used successfully for so long. Herbs contain various biochemical constituents—hormones, enzymes, vitamins, minerals, essential fatty acids, chlorophyll, fiber, and many other important elements. Herbs provide the body with vitamins, minerals, and other nutrients needed to boost the immune system and to aid the body in healing itself.

Herbs are most effective when used in their natural, balanced state. The body appears to be able to utilize herbs when and where they are needed and naturalists believe the body is readily able to receive and assimilate their nutrients. Herbs are different from drugs in that they almost always contain elements in the amounts that nature intended. Herbalists believe that the natural approach of using herbs can add health and vigor to the body because herbs provide a broad array of catalysts which work together synergistically and harmoniously, resulting in the complete healing of the body in most cases.

Drugs made synthetically from plants are no longer in their natural form and people often find that these drugs cause more harm than good because of side effects. In contrast, herbs are natural, safe and do not build up in the body producing side effects. There seem to be herbs that are of value to every system of the body. Still, herbs need to be used with wisdom and knowledge. They should not be used or mixed with other medications unless directed by a physician.

Single herbs do not always contain the proper healing qualities that are required for the symptoms being treated. Herbal combinations, however, are generally formulated to complement one another. By combining several herbs together, formulas are able to treat many symptoms that a single herb cannot. The following is a list of some of the herbs and natural nutrients that may be of benefit to those with fibromyalgia and other systemic conditions:

RED CLOVER

Red clover is a natural blood purifier and builder and is normally used in its liquid form. It is used to give the body energy and to protect and strengthen the immune system. This herb is high in vitamin A and is an excellent choice in any tea-blend as it is usually more effective when complemented with other herbs. Some of the herbs complementary to red clover are prickly ash bark, echinacea, cascara bark, rosemary, and buckthorn bark.

Research has indicated that red clover contains some antibiotic properties that are beneficial against bacteria. This herb has been used for treating bronchitis, cancer, nervous conditions, and removing toxins from the body. It is invaluable to the fibromyalgia sufferer because it is high in selenium, which is very important in the nutritional regimen, and because it also contains manganese, sodium, calcium, copper, and magnesium. Red clover contains vitamin C as well, necessary for boosting the immune system and disease prevention, and the B-complex vitamins.

PASSIONFLOWER

This herb has properties that are helpful for the nerves and circulation. Passionflower works well in formulas designed to treat insomnia and also works effectively in formulas designed to combat nervous tension, anxiety, stress, restlessness, and nervous headaches. Passionflower is helpful for fevers and is one of the more effective herbs for the nervous system.

VALERIAN

Valerian is probably the herb most widely used for anxiety and nervous tension. It is used as a natural sedative to improve the quality of sleep and relieve insomnia and is also used to combat depression. Valerian contains essential oils and alkaloids which reportedly combine to produce the calming, sedative effect. Considered a nervine herb, it is used as a very safe non-narcotic herbal sedative and has been used for after-pains in childbirth, heart palpitations, muscle spasms, and arthritis. Valerian is rich in calcium, which accounts for its ability to strengthen the spine, nerves, and brain. It is also high in magnesium, which works with calcium for healthy bones and the nervous system. It is also very high in selenium and manganese to strengthen the immune system and contains zinc and vitamins A and C.

CHAMOMILE

Chamomile possesses relaxing properties that prove to be very effective in promoting relaxation and inducing sleep. It is also promotes digestion and assists in assimilating nutrients from food, thereby enhancing metabolism and the utilization of energy. Ancient Egyptians used chamomile for its healing properties. Recent animals studies have proven chamomile to have antihistaminic effects along with anti-ulcer and antibacterial properties. It is useful for cleansing the liver, increasing mental alertness, promoting natural hormones, and for revitalizing the texture of skin and hair.

Chamomile is high in calcium and magnesium which strengthen the nervous system, promote restful sleep, and improve the strength of the immune system. It also contains vitamins A, C, F, and B-complex, making it effective for the nervous system. Selenium and zinc, significant for the immune system, are also found in chamomile. Finally, the herb contains tryptophan, the component that allows it to work as a sedative and promote sleep.

PAU D'ARCO

Pau d'arco is reported to be a natural blood cleanser and builder. It also possesses antibiotic properties which aid in destroying viral infections in the body. It helps combat cancer and has been used to strengthen the body, increase energy, and strengthen the immune system.

GINSENG

Ginseng is one of the oldest and most beneficial herbs in the world. Research has shown that the roots are effective against bronchitis and heart disease. Ginseng has also been found to reduce blood cholesterol, improve brain function and memory, increase physical stamina, stimulate the endocrine glands, strengthen the central nervous system, and build the immune system.

Ginseng has been rated as the most potent of herbs because it supports so many body functions. It benefits the heart and circulation, normalizes blood pressure, and prevents arteriosclerosis. It is also used to help protect the body against radiation and as an antidote to drugs and toxic chemicals.

Ginseng contains vitamin A and vitamin E, the component essential for a healthy heart and circulatory system. It also contains the B vitamins thiamine, riboflavin, B12, and niacin, all necessary for maintaining healthy nerves, hair, skin, eyes, and muscle tone. The minerals magnesium, iron, calcium, potassium, and manganese are also found in ginseng.

GOLDENSEAL

Goldenseal assists in boosting a sluggish glandular system and promoting hormone production. A very powerful nutrient that goes directly into the blood stream and assists in regulating liver function, goldenseal is reported to act as a natural form of insulin by providing the body with nutrients necessary to produce its own insulin. This aids metabolism and energy production and makes goldenseal a very effective nutrient for fibromyalgia. It is also reported to act as a natural antibiotic to stop infections.

Goldenseal contains the alkaloids hydrastine and hydrastinine that have strong astringent and antiseptic effects on mucus membranes. The antibiotic properties of goldenseal are largely due to its alkaloid content, including berberine, which has been found to be effective against organisms such as staphylococcus, streptococcus, salmonella, and *Candida albicans*. Goldenseal is a very powerful immune booster.

This herb contains vitamins A, C, E, F, and B-complex. It also contains potassium, phosphorus, iron, calcium, zinc, and manganese.

GOTU KOLA

Gotu kola is said to be a valuable treatment for depression by helping with mental fatigue and memory loss. Naturalists recommend gotu kola for rejuvenating the nervous system. It is sometimes referred to as "brain food" because of its ability to energize brain function. It is also used to increase circulation, neutralize blood toxins, help balance hormones, and relax the nerves.

Gotu kola is rich in magnesium and also contains vitamins A, C, and K which protect the lungs from disease and the immune system against diseases. Vitamin K is necessary for blood clotting and in healing colitis. Gotu kola is a good source of manganese, niacin, zinc, calcium, sodium, and vitamins B1 and B2.

ALOE VERA

Although the aloe vera plant looks like a cactus, it is actually a member of the lily family. Aloe vera is known to promote healing when used externally. It has also been used effectively for treating radiation burns. Also vera is known to help increase movement in the intestines, promote menstruation, relieve constipation, and aid in digestion. In this way it works to aid the body in eliminating toxins. Aloe has been used very effectively to assist with inflammation and ulcers. It can also help clean, soothe, and relieve pain. It contains salicylic acid and magnesium which function together as an analgesic.

Aloe vera is high in vitamin C and selenium, two powerful antioxidants that help prevent and cure diseases. It also contains vitamins A and B-complex, phosphorus, magnesium, potassium, niacin, manganese, and zinc.

ECHINACEA

Echinacea is a very powerful nutrient that stimulates the immune response in the body and assists the body in increasing its ability to resist infection. It also assists in the promotion of white blood cells and is helpful as a blood purifier. Echinacea is considered a natural antibiotic. Echinacea was used by the native Americans for snake bites, insect stings, and infections. Extracts of echinacea root have been found to contain interferon-like properties. Interferon is produced naturally in the body to prevent viral infections and has been known to fight chemical toxic poisoning in the body.

Echinacea contains vitamin C which helps to promote healing and fights infections. Calcium and vitamin E are also found in this powerful herb. Echinacea contains iodine which assists the thyroid gland in regulating metabolism, mental development, and energy production. It also contains potassium for muscle contraction, kidney function, and nerve function. The sulfur content of echinacea helps to dissolve acids in the body and improve circulation.

SLIPPERY ELM

Slippery elm is a demulcent which buffers against irritations and inflammations of the mucous membranes. A very powerful nutrient for fibromyalgia sufferers, it also helps to assist the activity of the adrenal glands and is a nutritious herb for both internal and external healing. It has been used primarily to treat stomach and intestinal ulcers, gastrointestinal problems, digestion acidity, and to lubricate the bowels. Slippery elm is also a blood builder and a supporter of the cardiovascular system. It is equal to oatmeal in vitamin and mineral content.

Slippery elm contains vitamins A, K, F, and P, all important in building and toning the lungs, stomach, and colon. Minerals contained in slippery elm are selenium, copper, zinc, iron, calcium, phosphorus, and potassium.

ROSEMARY

Rosemary is of great benefit in replacing aspirin for the treatment of headaches. This unique herb assists in combating stress and improving memory. It is very high in calcium and is considered of benefit to the entire nervous system.

HERBAL TEAS

There are a number of delicious herbal teas that are excellent alternatives to soft drinks (normally loaded with sugar) and bottled fruit juices (usually contain considerable amounts of fructose). Try herbal teas such as chamomile, spearmint, peppermint, cinnamon, orange peel, and valerian root. You can drink the tea hot or chilled or you can make it into popsicles by pouring it into molds and freezing. A calming and soothing combination tea for help in inducing sleep is passionflower, valerian, hops, and chamomile. Take the tea half an hour before bed. Green herbal teas are especially helpful particularly for strengthening the immune system.

Other Supplements

APPLE CIDER VINEGAR

Apple cider vinegar is known as one of the best total body purifiers and cleansers. It is most effective when used in its organic form. It is usually a very potent formula and is best tolerated mixed with a healthy juice or purified water.

MELATONIN

In the 1950s scientists discovered melatonin, a hormone which may be the partial answer to sleep problems. It may also may have the capability to affect other common distresses such as lack of immunity, aging, and cancer. Melatonin is produced by a small gland found in the center of the brain, the pineal gland. The pineal gland releases melatonin when the eye is not receiving light. Melatonin controls our sleep cycles and helps us to rest soundly. Another tremendous benefit of melatonin is that it contains vitamin E, one of the more powerful antioxidants and free radical fighters.

MALIC ACID

Malic acid is a food supplement found in citrus fruits and apples. Studies have found that it assists energy, metabolism, and production of muscle energy. When combined with magnesium, malic acid is a very powerful aid for the fibromyalgia sufferer.

PYCNOGENOL (PROANTHOCYANADINS)

Pycnogenol is a substance produced from grape seed extract and maritime pine bark that has been determined by scientists to be 50 times stronger than vitamin E. Its primary function is that of a very powerful antioxidant which scavenges free radicals generated by foreign toxic chemicals. It has also been thought to help remove inflammation from the joints and other tissues as well as improving the nervous and immune systems. Beyond that, pycnogenol strengthens collagen, improves circulation, enhances the permeability of cell walls, acts as a powerful antioxidant to boost the immune system, enhances metabolism, and promotes healing in the body.

RICE BRAN EXTRACT

Scientists have reportedly found that three of the tocotryonols in the polyphenols of rice bran carry a form of vitamin E that is 6,000 times stronger than the current forms of vitamin E. Vitamin E is a powerful antioxidant and helps with capillary wall strength, lung metabolism, muscle and nerve maintenance, and acts as an immune booster and detoxifier.

COENZYME Q-10

The discovery of coenzyme Q-10 is of tremendous benefit to mankind. It compares with vitamins A, C, and E as a powerful antioxidant. Research is supporting the fact that CoQ-10 benefits diseases associated with nutrient deficiencies such as cancer, aging, heart disease, obesity, and now fibromyalgia. This nutrient aids in the oxygenation of cells and tissues. It is found in food sources such as spinach, sardines, and peanuts. CoQ-10, estimated to be 20 times stronger than vitamin E and is considered to boost biochemical ability and activate cellular energy while improving circulation. One research study found that CoQ-10 literally doubled the immune system's ability to clear invading organisms from the blood.

DHEA (DEHYDROEPIANDOSTERONE)

DHEA, an adrenal hormone, is the most abundant hormone in the body and is often considered "the mother hormone." It is a precursor to the sex hormones as well as a number of other vital hormones in the body. Levels of DHEA are the highest when we are in the prime of life (age 20-35). DHEA is now available without prescription and has great value in preventing and treating osteoporosis, diabetes, cancer, Alzheimer's, cardiovascular disease, high cholesterol, and other immune disorders such as chronic fatigue syndrome and fibromyalgia. It is also thought to be effective in reducing the symptoms of PMS and menopause. It is sometimes called the "miracle" hormone because it is believed to slow down and even reverse the aging process. When recommended nutrients are ingested to boost and balance the bodily systems, then DHEA will be produced naturally and more readily in the body.

L-CARNITINE

L-carnitine is an amino acid which assists greatly in breaking down fats and sugars for energy in the metabolic process. It is very effective with the fibromyalgia patient for raising energy levels.

BEE POLLEN

Bee pollen is very high in protein and considered one of the most complete foods that we can consume. It contains vitamins, minerals, amino acids, proteins, enzymes, and fats. It helps when there is a hormone imbalance in the body. Bee pollen is very useful to fibromyalgia patients because it helps to increase appetite, normalize intestinal activity, strengthen capillary walls, offset the effects of drugs and pollutants, and is one of the most powerful immune boosters known to man.

GLUCOSAMINE

Glucosamine is the key substance that determines how many proteoglycan (water holding) molecules are formed in cartilage. It has been found very effective for improvement in arthritic conditions. Also, in a study conducted by the Vulvodynia Project, glucosamine was used to effectively reduce sensitivity and pain in soft tissue areas of fibromyalgia patients.

CHONDROITIN SULFATES

Chondroitin sulfates are naturally occurring substances that inhibit enzymes that can degrade cartilage. At the same time it helps to attract fluid to the proteoglycan molecules.

CHAPTER 9

An Arthritis Review

Arthritis attacks one in six Americans, totaling approximately 50,000,000 people with the condition (Mankin, 1994). It attacks individuals of all ages and both sexes, but the percentages do indicate that more women are generally afflicted than are men, as is the case with fibromyalgia. The distinction between fibromyalgia and arthritis should be made here. Although both are certainly systemic conditions, fibromyalgia is a debilitating connective tissue and muscular condition, while the more common forms of arthritis are a result of free radical damage and inflammation in the joints. It has been documented that inflammation is not a characteristic of fibromyalgia.

The term arthritis refers to over one hundred conditions that affect the bones, joints, muscles, and connective tissue. It is also important to note that not all joint pains are arthritis. There are many self–limiting conditions, especially viral infections, such as mononucleosis and flu that may cause transient joint pain. Therefore, it is important that some of the chronic types of arthritis not be diagnosed until the symptoms are present for six to eight weeks or longer. The more common symptoms of arthritis are pain and stiffness and it can be a very frustrating disease since it is so nebulous and keeps the medical professional, health professionals, and even the patient guessing. For example, an individual may awaken in the early morning stiff and in pain and in the course of the day gradually be pain free and have more free movement, only to be assaulted again before the end of the day. One general guideline in diagnosing arthritis is if a morning stiffness and pain characterized by an inflammation lasts more than 30 minutes.

To confuse the issue even further, stress, emotional upset, and changes in the weather may also be responsible for day to day fluctuations with arthritic conditions. Due to these conditions and fluctuations, activity should be generally observed for long periods of time and even trends charted to thoroughly diagnose the condition of arthritis. To add more to the mystery are the behavioral aspects of arthritis. It may fluctuate in totality, just as it fluctuates on a daily basis. For example, a spontaneous remission can occur with an arthritic patient where they might experience a complete absence of symptoms for days, weeks, and months, and in some rare cases a fortunate individual may see arthritis move out for good (Rooney & Rooney, 1986).

The underlying cause of arthritis is unknown. Many physicians and practitioners will also tell you that it is incurable and that arthritis patients and victims will simply have to learn to live with it. In 1970, the Arthritis Foundation took an official position that there was no special diet for arthritis and that there was no official treatment other than drug therapy and surgery. Today the Arthritis Foundation and the medical professionals are looking into the question of how diet might affect the immune system. However, both are still supporting the fact that it is too early to recommend any special diet or special treatment.

Let us look more at what arthritis really is, its cause, and its actual condition. *Arthritis* really means "inflammation of the joint." The term itself has sort of become a "catch all" term to describe any ache or pain. Casual exercisers, like those who go to aerobics, those who play softball or other sports on the weekends, may have a temporary inflammation of the joints. Also, flu, colds, and viruses can upset the body's hormonal balance and cause a temporary inflammation in the joints, but we certainly do not say or indicate that it is incurable. In fact, the body repairs such injuries quite well. On a more long term or chronic basis, such as with age, many people fail to keep up with the damage and develop pain in their joints as a result of aging and wear and tear. The wearing and tearing is normally called osteoarthritis and it is precisely what most people have when they say they have arthritis, this being the most common type of arthritis.

The joints that carry the most weight are the hips, knees, and the lower back, and this is normally where pain is the most common. Basically your leg joint cartilage bears all your weight and does not have all of its bone supply. Small wonder that this is one of the first bodily systems that give out. Thus, the massive number of knee and hip joint replacements in our society today.

It is very significant that arthritis is an inflammatory disease. It is a known medical fact that when a part of the body is inflamed (including the joints) that your immune system bombards it with free radicals. This toxic shower of free radicals is a plus within the body's immune system. It is one of the ways your body kills off invading microbes like flue and/or other viruses. Your immune system produces its own free radicals consistently by the billions. In the case of an injured joint, however, this body response can be inappropriate in that it actually adds to the confusion and problem, being a chain reaction and/or an auto-immune response that can attack the body, and the body ends up fighting and damaging itself with an inappropriate flooding of the free radicals. The result of this is serious damage to the joints. In fact, such a free radical attack can break down membranes, cartilage, and disrupt the production of your synovial fluid. One particular renowned researcher/rheumatologist states that an autoimmune inflammatory response has a tendency to feed on itself. Like an atomic reactor accelerating out of control, the first inflammatory interactions beget later ones in a cycle that is very hard to break, and if the inflammation lasts too long, the collateral damage becomes too great for the body. The second most common form of arthritis, rheumatoid arthritis, is a result of this extreme form of an autoimmune response. Fortunately, this debilitating type of arthritis, affects fewer people, about 7 million. However, it does attack the whole body at once and is a more serious condition than osteoarthritis. It appears that arthritis tends to occur when your immune system makes a mistake and attacks your body's normal tissues with a bombardment of a detrimental array of free radicals. It appears that this occurrence is a result of one of five things, but certainly other causative factors could exist:

1. Lack of good nutrition
2. Lack of proper supplements and antioxidants
3. Lack of exercise
4. Undue stress, anxiety, and depression (lack of good stress management skills)
5. Injury

Precautions when Treating Arthritis

As with stroke, cancer, and heart disease, traditional treatment of arthritis has included drugs and surgery. True to form, these treatments are short ranged, stop gaps and on the long haul the condition will normally worsen due to the breakdown of the immune system as a side effect of the drugs.

The past traditional medical approach has been an effort to relieve pain with drugs that only mask the pain. We have traditionally treated the symptoms with medication without getting to the cause, and making things much worse because of a battery of side effects.

Traditional Treatments

Medications typically used for arthritis pain relief are NSAIDS (nonsteroidal anti-inflammatory drugs) that typically include ibuprofen (i.e., Advil, Nuprin, or Motrin). NSAIDS can cause gastrointestinal bleeding and deplete iron levels, problems that most people usually aren't even aware of. Anyone taking NSAIDs should look for a good multivitamin with at least 18 mg of iron—not exceeding that without their physician's approval.

Arthritis patients also typically take several aspirins a day. It is common knowledge that aspirin in excess can cause bleeding of the stomach and may even cause ulcers. Aspirin also depresses the immune system and sets the individual up for more illnesses.

Arthritis victims in many cases ask for cortisone shots in an attempt to obtain relief from arthritis symptoms. Cortisone-like drugs are called corticosteroids with side effects such as cataracts, bone loss (which leads to osteoporosis), diabetes, high blood pressure, and a breakdown of the immune system on a long term basis. Corticosteroids put bones at risk for osteoporosis by blocking calcium absorption and interfering with vitamin D. The arthritic patient should consider bolstering their calcium intake with calcium supplements to reach recommended levels. Women over fifty and men over sixty-five years of age need a total of about 1500 mg of calcium a day. All others need approximately 1,000 mg a day. Also, an addition of 400 I.U. of vitamin D should be taken in a multi-vitamin type supplement and the arthritic patient should ask their physician to monitor their bone density. (See Chapter 5 for the correct dosages of other vitamins, minerals and nutrients needed.)

Important Points Concerning Arthritis

- It is critical to stop the process of arthritis and free radical damage early, if possible. If not reversed early, permanent damage can occur and can become very difficult to reverse.
- Low impact/mild exercise is critically important because the physical movements of the joints squeeze out waste and permit the cartilage to take in nutrients. It is very important on a daily basis to move every joint in the body in every direction they are created to move in. (See Chapter 6 on exercise.)
- Make a lifestyle change nutritionally and utilize the 21-day detoxification/nutrition program found in Chapter 5. Once you have assisted the body in detoxing nutritionally to get the poisons out, then follow the "Now What after 21 days" nutritional program in Chapter 5 for a lifestyle change.
- Complete the stress analysis in chapter 7 to discover the areas in your life that are impacting you and causing you the most stress. Then follow the well designed stress management program that follows your stress analysis as a lifestyle change.
- Take the proper nutritional supplements, including the power nutrients and antioxidants (outlined in Chapter 5) to boost the body's immune system so that inappropriate free radical attacks may be managed more efficiently.

THE VARIOUS TYPES OF ARTHRITIS

There are more than 100 types of arthritis, but I will discuss only the more common types of arthritis that affect the majority of the population (Rooney and Rooney, 1986).

Osteoarthritis

Osteoarthritis is the most common type and, with the aging process, the form of arthritis most people are likely to experience. It is also referred to as "degenerative joint disease." There are at least two kinds of osteoarthritis referred to generally as primary and secondary.

Primary osteoarthritis is very often more prevalent in the small joints of the body, such as the hands. Secondary osteoarthritis very often develops after an injury or when there is repeated strain in a joint that may have been previously damaged. It is not uncommon for a person to develop more than one type of arthritis. For instance, it is very common for one to have rheumatoid arthritis while at the same experiencing osteoarthritis.

Secondary osteoarthritis most often appears in the larger joints, such as the hips, spine, and the knees. Pain is generally the most common symptom of osteoarthritis and it can be generally relieved with rest. There is usually swelling, a warm feeling, and also stiffness when there is associated inflammation. With osteoarthritis there are "creaking or grating" sounds given off when the joint is in use. A brief description of osteoarthritis includes the fact that damage generally starts in the cartilage that covers the bones. With the aging process, over a period of time, the cartilage wears down and tends to lose its smooth surface. Eventually, the underlying bones (the bones under the cartilage) harden and form bony spurs, causing rough, irregular surfaces that rub against each other.

Rheumatoid Arthritis

Inflammation also plays a major role in rheumatoid arthritis and interestingly enough, not only in the joints, but also in the muscles as well as the heart, lungs, eyes and even in the nervous system. The inflammation usually begins in the synovium, which is the thin membrane that lines the joints. The synovium becomes thickened and eventually invades the cartilage and then later the bone. This is the cause of major joint damage over a long period of time. Normally, in rheumatoid arthritis, the smaller joints of the feet, wrists, elbows, shoulders, hands, and knees are involved. The symptoms of rheumatoid arthritis usually come on very gradually, however, in about 10 percent of the cases, the onset is very abrupt, almost overnight in some cases. Rheumatoid arthritis affects almost 3 percent of the general population, it may occur at any age, and about 75 percent of those affected are women. The common symptoms of rheumatoid arthritis are excessive fatigue, prolonged stiffness, especially in the morning, and pain in joints at rest and in use. A weight loss, slight fever, and loss of appetite may also occur.

Finally, the prognosis, or the future outlook, for arthritis is very much misunderstood. Most people hold the belief that rheumatoid arthritis is a universally crippling disease. At present, with better diagnosis and improved treatment, including all natural treatment regimens (such as the book you are now reading), only about 5 percent or less of those developing rheumatoid arthritis will develop deformities severe enough to restrict them to a bed or a wheelchair. With the new, natural advances and promising research, there is very good reason to hope that the cause, and ultimately the cure, for rheumatoid arthritis will be found.

Gout

Gout is generally due to excessive deposits of uric acid crystals in the joint. Uric acid is a very normal substance in the body; however, increased amounts can be caused by: hereditary factors, obesity, diuretic pills, excessive alcohol, and the kidney's lack of ability to rid the body of excessive uric acid.

Gout can affect any joint but it generally settles in the leg or the foot. The characteristic of the affected joint is that it becomes very hot and swollen and very tender to the touch. Unlike some other forms of arthritis, gout usually comes on very acutely, even overnight, and the pain is just as immediate and just as severe as the gradual onset of the chronic types of arthritis. The treatment of gout may require removing fluid from an affected joint and observing it under a microscope to check for uric acid crystals. An elevated uric acid level itself is not specific, meaning that a person with an elevated uric acid level will not necessarily develop gout.

Ankylosing Spondylitis

Ankylosing spondylitis typically affects men and women equally. Although men tend to have more symptoms, women tend to have a milder form of the disease and one that more frequently involves peripheral joints such as the hip and the knee. Stiffness and lower back pain are the more common symptoms that have the tendency to come and go while the stiffness often gets better with low impact type exercise. The normal course of the condition can vary greatly, but it often progresses slowly leading to a fusion of the spine and a loss of flexibility.

Systemic Lupus Erythematosus

This is commonly known or referred to as lupus or SLE. Lupus is often characterized by inflammation of many of the internal organs and it may also occur as a skin rash, chest pain, joint pain, fever, kidney problems, anemia, and even neuralgic problems such as seizures. In other words, lupus can masquerade in many different forms, therefore it is very difficult for a physician or a practitioner to make an accurate diagnosis.

The diagnosis of lupus is normally made in a physician's office following a physical, several different types of laboratory tests, and an examination of the patient's history. A person with lupus will indicate several abnormalities including low white blood and platelet count, elevated SED rate, anemia, protein and red blood cells in the urine, and a positive antinuclear antibody (ANA). The ANA although nonspecific, remains the best screening test for lupus.

Although the cause of lupus remains unknown, much of the evidence and research suggests that female sex hormones (estrogen), one's genetic background, and environmental background are all involved. A final note, the disease of lupus affects women normally about five times more often than men and it usually strikes between the ages of 20 and 40, although it can occur at any age.

Bursitis

Bursitis is inflammation of the bursa surrounding the joints and is very often confused with arthritis of the joints. The bursa is a sac of fluid which allows muscles and tendons to move around the joint. Bursitis most frequently affects the shoulders, hips, and elbows. One of the signs and symptoms of bursitis is significant swelling and redness of the bursa sac, which helps explain why it is confused with arthritis of the joints. A physician can diagnose bursitis upon physical examination by localizing points of tenderness outside the joints, indicating that it is the bursa sac rather than the joint itself. Results of lab tests are usually normal.

Back Pain

Back pain is a very common symptom of many different types of arthritis. However, arthritis is certainly not the only cause of back pain. Other causes are lack of exercise, emotional upset, posture problems, and congenital malformations of the spine. Osteoarthritis is the most common form of arthritis that causes chronic low back pain. Bone spurs and disc degeneration from osteoarthritis will compress the muscles as they exit the spinal canal. Other forms of arthritis that cause low back pain are ankylosing spondylitis, psoriatic arthritis, rheumatoid arthritis, and Reiter's syndrome. Pain in the back can originate from the vertebrae, ligaments, muscles, discs (which are the cushions between vertebrae), and the nerves. Some of the common problems that cause back pain include obesity and lack of exercise, which puts a great deal of stress on the muscles which are essential to support the spine. Also, injuries from athletics, accidents, and awkward movements during routine activities can injure muscles, ligaments, and discs causing low back pain.

Reiter's Syndrome

The cause of Reiter's syndrome is unknown. However, it has been known to onset after particular infections of the bowel or urethra. The most frequent victims of Reiter's syndrome are primarily young men between the ages of 20 and 40; however, women can also contract the disease.

The diagnosis of Reiter's syndrome is generally made in a physician's office after a physical examination, laboratory tests, and a personal history. There is not a specific test for diagnosing Reiter's, but the rheumatoid factor is negative, there may be mild anemia, and the SED (Sedimentation Erythrocyte) rate is usually elevated. The SED is a common blood test that physicians can perform in their office and it will indicate how active certain types of arthritis are, including rheumatoid arthritis and it is a method of determining the activity of inflammation in the body.

Juvenile Rheumatoid Arthritis (JRA)

Somewhere between 50,000 and 200,000 children suffer from JRA. Other forms of arthritis that affect children are ankylosing spondylitis and systemic lupus erythematosus or SLE. Girls are generally affected more than boys; however, the ratio seems to vary with age and presentation of the disease. The effects of JRA may include enlargement of the spleen and lymph nodes, inflammation of the eyes and even growth retardation. Severe pain when a child is at rest is very unusual which is in contrast to adult rheumatoid .arthritis.

Juvenile rheumatoid arthritis offers its first signs sometimes with a child limping because of limited motion in a knee or an ankle.

A physician's diagnosis of JRA is often very difficult at first because many other different conditions need to be eliminated. Laboratory tests, however, will usually reveal anemia, a negative rheumatoid factor, an elevated SED rate, and finally x-rays of the involved joints most often are normal. Most rheumatologists and physicians report that the overall outlook or prognosis for JRA is very favorable. Seventy-five to ninety percent of children with JRA have a good prognosis with no symptoms or only mild ones with little or no deformity.

Regular eye examinations by an ophthalmologist are a good idea so as to detect early inflammation of the eyes (iritis), since it very often occurs without symptoms and is very treatable. Regular conferences with family members, physicians, and even teachers are suggested so that the child can understand and cope with this disease more effectively.

Raynaud's Phenomenon

This phenomenon is quite common and generally affects young women between the ages of twenty to forty years. In many cases people will have Raynaud's for many years and not develop any other condition. However, some may develop another form of arthritis after Raynaud's, sometimes systemic lupus erythematosus and especially scleroderma (hardening of the skin). Raynaud's phenomenon generally occurs with cold weather exposure. The color of the skin changes from white to blue or red. The treatment of Raynaud's is generally involved with protecting the fingers and hands from the cold and always wearing gloves in cold weather. Raynaud's phenomenon may appear as symptoms of burning, tingling fingertips, or ulcers on the tips of the fingers.

Sjogren's Syndrome

This syndrome is an autoimmune condition that is generally characterized or manifested by chronic inflammation of the salivary and lachrymal glands (tear producing). The inflammation in Sjogren's syndrome will gradually damage these glands, causing a decreased production of saliva and tears, which results in dry mouth and dry eyes.

About 15 percent of those with rheumatoid arthritis will have Sjogren's syndrome. It may also occur with systemic lupus erythematosus. Sjogren's can occur as a primary condition, meaning that it is without any other type of arthritis, or that it is not stimulated by any other condition, or it may occur as a secondary condition, most commonly associated with rheumatoid arthritis.

Sjogren's syndrome may be associated with other autoimmune conditions that affect the body such as neurologic conditions, thyroid disorders, and conditions of the stomach and bile, and finally diseases that affect the hormone glands. In the diagnosis of Sjogren's syndrome, laboratory tests may reveal anemia, a positive rheumatoid factor, an elevated SED rate, and elevated serum proteins.

APPENDIX A: EXAMPLE DAILY LOG

Date __Th. 3/17__

NUTRITION

Bkfst.	Snack	Lunch	Snack	Dinner	Snack	Comments
whole wheat toast oatmeal w/honey o.J. & coffee	whole wheat bagel	fish baked potato peach water	veggies and dip	chicken rice vegetable salad angel food cake	apple bran flakes w/skim milk	Enjoying eating again — my energy is increasing I love it!!

EXERCISE

Aerobics	Strength	Flexibility
walked for 23 minutes (a.m.)	worked out — with Body Advantage 20 minutes (afternoon)	

STRESS COPING

Mental	Physical	Emotional
read a novel for 45 min.	foot massage hot shower	talked to Joey

MEDICATIONS/NUTRIENTS

Drugs/Nutrients	Dosage	Time
aspirin	3	7 a.m.
colloidal minerals	2 oz.	8 a.m.
multi-vitamin	6 caps.	8 am./6 p.m.

WHAT TO ASK OR CONSULT WITH MY PHYSICIAN ABOUT

I haven't taken anti-depressants for 3 weeks — if I continue w/herbs & vitamins can I stay off them?

DAILY DIARY

Had a good day! Headaches are gone — not so sore after exercise. Beginning to sleep better.

Daily Record (1-10) 10 being severe Pain __6__ Stiffness __4__ Irritability __5__

GLOSSARY OF TERMS

Acetaminophen: A pain-relieving and fever-reducing drug used in many over-the-counter drugs.

Acupuncture: An ancient Chinese healing art that involves inserting very thin needles into certain points along the body to relieve pain and promote healing.

Acupressure: Application of pressure over specific muscle sites to relieve pain and muscle spasm.

Acute: Begins quickly and is intense or sharp; sharp or severe.

Aerobic: designating activities involving increased oxygen consumption by the body as a result of aerobic exercise and/or exercises involving the legs, i.e., cycling, swimming, and walking.

Acupressure: Application of pressure over specific muscle sites to relieve pain and muscle spasm.

Anaphylaxis: A rare, severe allergic reaction characterized by difficulty in breathing or swelling, a swollen tongue, dizziness, fainting, hives, puffy eyelids, fast and irregular heartbeat or pulse, and/or a change in face color.

Anemia: A reduction to below normal in the number of red blood cells in the blood. A common symptom of anemia is fatigue.

Ankylosing spondylitis: A type of arthritis that primarily affects the spine and sacroiliac joints. Tendons and ligaments may become inflamed where they attach to the bone. Advanced forms may result in the formation of bony bridges between vertebrae, causing the spine to become rigid.

Antibody: A type of blood protein made by the body in response to a foreign substance (antigen). An antibody binds to an antigen and eliminates it from the body.

Antidepressant: A medication utilized in relief of depression or the blues, tricyclic antidepressants help to relieve night-time muscle spasms in fibromyalgia victims.

Antigen: Any substance the body regards as foreign or potentially dangerous, and that results in the production of an antibody.

Antihistamine: Inhibits or counteracts the action of histamine, a biological chemical produced in immune response. Histamine has a powerful effect, i.e., dilating blood vessels and the stimulation of the secretion of gastric juices. These drugs can also cause drowsiness, a serious problem for people with fibromyalgia who are battling stress and fatigue.

Anti-inflammatory drug: A drug, such as aspirin or ibuprofen, that reduces pain, redness, swelling and heat.

Antinuclear antibody test (ANA): A screening test used for several types of inflammatory conditions, and especially useful in detecting systemic lupus erythematosus. It is positive antinuclear antibodies may also be formed in reaction to certain medications, viral infections, liver diseases, various types of arthritis and even aging.

Apnea (Sleep): The hesitation or stopping of breathing during sleep, caused by obstructions within the nasal airway, sometimes occurring a multiple number of times during the night. This condition is also very closely associated with obesity, although not all obese people have sleep apnea. The brain must arouse the sleeper from deep sleep to relieve the obstruction and restore breathing, therefore, sleep apnea has serious health effects such as with the fibromyalgia sufferer.

Arthrodesis: Fixing a joint through surgery to relieve pain or give support; fusion.

Arthroscope: A flexible viewing tube about the diameter of a pencil, inserted through a small incision into the joint capsule, that provides a view of the inside of a joint.

Arthrosopic surgery: Surgery done on a joint using an arthroscope.

Articular: Refers to a joint. (More broadly, it means "the place of junction between two discrete objects.")

Atrophy: Decrease in size of a normally developed organ or tissue; wasting.

Autoimmune disease: A disease due to the action of the immune system against itself, occurring because the immune cells can't differentiate between the body's own material ("self") and that which is foreign ("non-self"). It is possible that certain body proteins are so altered by viral infections, by combination with a drug or chemical, or by extensive trauma, that they are no longer recognizable by the body as "self" and therefore are rejected as foreign.

Biofeedback: A procedure utilizing equipment to monitor the heart rate, skin temperature, muscle tension, and blood pressure. These body signals are exhibited on a monitor or screen so that one can observe how the body is responding. This process or procedure makes one more aware of a reaction to stress and/or pain and to assist the educational process of learning to control the body's physical and emotional reactions.

Biological: A laboratory-concocted agent, similar to the body's own biochemicals and administered in the same manner as drugs, that alters the body's immune response.

Bone spur: A bony growth around the joints seen in people with osteoarthritis. Joints may appear to be swollen.

Bursa: A small sac surrounding the joint and/or located between a tendon and bone. The bursae provide lubrication and reduce friction for joint movement.

Bursitis: Inflammation of the bursas, small, fluid-filled sacs that cushion and reduce friction where muscles and tendons move over bones or ligaments, such as in the shoulders, hips, knees, and elbows.

Carpal tunnel syndrome: A group of symptoms resulting from compression of the medial nerve in the wrist, with pain and burning or tingling numbness in the fingers and hand, sometimes extending to the elbow.

Cartilage: A smooth, resilient tissue that covers the ends of the bones so they don't' rub against each other.

Chondroitin sulfate: A product available in some health-food stores that contains glycosaminoglycans, major structural components of cartilage and connective tissue. Although this product is popular in Europe, there are no good U.S. studies to show it helps rebuild cartilage.

Chromosome: A structure in the nucleus of every cell containing genetic material that determines the characteristics of the cell.

Chronic: Persisting for a long time.

Chronic Fatigue Syndrome (CFS): A condition manifesting fatigue on a long term basis. The symptoms of CFS and fibromyalgia are almost identical with the only difference being the degree of pain that is characteristic in fibromylagia.

Chronobiology: This is the study of rhythms, cycles, and timing of biological events such as secretion of hormones, ovulation, and temperature fluctuations.

Circadian Rhythms: The daily, weekly, monthly, and seasonal schedules on which biological or living things carry out essential tasks such as eating, eliminating, digesting, and growing. Disruption of these rhythms occurs when, for instance, one travels across time zones. This can have a negative and sometimes profound impact on human performance and mood swings.

Clinical ecologist: An allergist with a special interest in environmental influences on health. More commonly known as an environmental physician.

Colchicine: A drug used in the treatment of gout, usually effective in terminating an attack of gout. Side effects may include gastrointestinal symptoms and low blood pressure.

Collagen vascular disease: An autoimmune disease in which the body's fibrous collagen tissues and the cells lining the inside of blood vessels overgrow, causing organ dysfunction and circulation problems.

Complete blood count (CBC): A diagnostic test that measures blood components, including white blood cells, red blood cells and platelets.

Computerized axial tomographic scan (a CT or CAT scan): A sophisticated x-ray imaging technique that produces thin cross-sectional images of body organs.

Connective tissue: a long-fiber type of body tissue that supports and connects internal organs, forms bones and the walls of blood vessels, attaches muscles to bone, and replaces tissues of other types following injury.

Corticosteroids: Hormones produced by the body and closely related to cortisone. Corticosteroids can be synthetically produced and have powerful anti-inflammatory effects. Prednisone and cortisone are two of the synthetic drugs produced by pharmaceutical companies.

Cortisone (corticosteroid): Potent and effective steroid drug related to the hormone cortisol, produced by the adrenal glands. Steroid drugs quickly reduce swelling and inflammation, bud do have possible serious side effects.

Culture: The propagation of microorganisms or living tissue in a special medium conducive to their growth. Fluid withdrawn from a joint might be cultured to see what microorganisms, if any, it contains.

Cyclosporine: A drug used to prevent rejection in organ-transplant patients, used with some success in people with rheumatoid arthritis who haven't responded well to other treatments.

Cyst: An enclosed sac or capsule in the body that contains fluid or a semisolid material. Although harmless, a cyst can become infected.

Deep heat: A treatment that uses tissue-penetrating ultrasound waves to heat up small areas of the body. This is the only heat treatment that can penetrate beyond the surface layers of the skin to a joint.

Degenerative joint disease: Osteoarthritis.

Delta Sleep: The deep, restorative, replenishing sleep required for many of the vital body functions such as antibody productions and restorative immune functioning. Disturbances of delta sleep are characteristic of fibromyalgia. The delta waves are brain waves produced during this very deep restorative sleep.

Depression: A state of mind characterized by feelings of worthlessness, irritability, loss of interest in normal activities, lack of sleep, anxiety, low self-esteem, dejection, sadness, and in some cases can be characterized with a preoccupation with loss, pain, death, or other unpleasant themes.

Discoid lupus: A form of lupus that affects only the skin, causing a rash usually across the face and upper part of the body.

Disease-modifying: Altering, changing or slowing the course of a disease.

DMSO *(dimethyl sulfoxide):* A solvent, unproven to work, that is sometimes applied to swollen, painful joints.

Echocardiogram: A test that uses sound waves to detect fluid around the heart and other heart abnormalities.

Eicosapentaenoic acid (EPA): Omega-3 fatty acids, found in fish such as mackerel, sardines and salmon, and shown to inhibit inflammation in the body.

Environmental physician: A doctor with a special interest in the impact that environment—air, water, food, toxins—has on the health of an individual. These doctors were formerly called clinical ecologists.

Erythrocyte sedimentation rate (*see* SED Rate): A test that measures how fast red blood cells cling together, fall and settle to the bottom of a test tube. The more inflammatory proteins found in the blood, the faster these cells clump together and sink.

Fibromylagia: A common clinical syndrome of generalized musculoskelatal pain, stiffness, and chronic aching characterized by reproducible tenderness on palpation of specific anatomical sites, generally referred to as tender pints. This systemic condition is considered primary when not associated with systemic cause such as trauma, cancer, thyroid disease and pathologies of rheumatic arthritis or connective tissues. The name fibromyalgia has for the most part replaced the term "fibrositis" which was once used to describe the disorder when there was suspicion that inflammation was a part of the fibromylagia condition.

Fibrous: Composed of or containing fibers. (e.g. Ligaments are rubbery bands of strong fibrous tissue.)

Flare-up: A period of time when symptoms worsen.

Gamma-interferon: A medicinal preparation derived from live cells that is being tried experimentally in the treatment of RA and other rheumatic diseases. A biochemical produced by certain of the body's immune cells, gamma-interferon has a range of effect on the body's immune system.

Gamma-linolenic acid (GLA): A fatty acid—found in high concentrations in black-current oil, evening-primrose oil, and borage oil—thought to have anti-inflammatory actions in the body.

Genetic markers: Specific genes or groups of genes on chromosomes that indicate a particular genetic tendency, including a tendency to develop certain types of diseases.

Glycosaminoglycans: Major structural components of cartilage and connective tissue. Available as chondroitin sulfate.

Gold salts: Gold compounds, given by injection or orally, used in the treatment of rheumatoid arthritis.

Gout: A form of arthritis caused by deposits of uric acid crystals in the joint. Gout usually strikes a single joint, often the big toe and often with sudden, severe pain.

Hematocrit: The volume percentage of red blood cells in whole blood.

Hemoglobin: A protein that transports oxygen in the blood.

Hemorrhage: The escape of blood from a ruptured vessel. Hemorrhage can be external, internal or into the skin or other tissues.

Hydroxy chloroquine: An antimalarial drug (brand name Plaquenil) that is used to treat rheumatoid arthritis.

Hypothalamic-Pituitary-Thyroid Axis: The primary brain-hormonal energy production response axes (i.e., the place where brain function and hormonal function are coordinated in response to the need for energy production).

Ibuprofen: A nonsteroid anti-inflammatory agent.

Immunosuppressive: Inhibiting the immune system in a way that interferes with the formation of antibodies.

Immunotoxin: A monoclonal antibody that contains a toxin. The antibody kills a targeted immune cell and thus represses inflammation.

Infectious arthritis: A type of arthritis caused by an infection somewhere in the body. The infection travels to the joint.

Inflammation: The body's protective response to an injury or infection. The classic signs—heat, redness, swelling and pain—are produced as a result of biochemicals secreted by the body's infection-fighting immune cells as they attempt to wall off and destroy any germs, and to break down and remove damaged tissue.

Joint capsule: A tough, fibrous, fluid-filled tissue that completely surrounds a joint. Synovial cells lining the joint capsule secrete fluid that keeps the joint lubricated.

Juvenile rheumatoid arthritis: Any type of arthritis that develops in children. There are several subtypes.

Ligament: A thick, cordlike fiber that attaches to bones to keep them in correct alignment.

Liver biopsy: A surgical procedure that removes a bit of liver tissue for examination. The tissue is procured using a long, hollow-core needle, which is inserted through the skin into the liver.

Lupus: See systemic lupus erythematosus.

Lyme disease: A type of arthritis caused by bacteria transmitted by a tick that infests a variety of animals, including deer, mice and domestic animals such as dogs.

Lymphoma: Cancer of the lymph glands, which are part of the immune system.

Magnetic resonance imaging (MRI): A noninvasive medical procedure that can produce images of soft tissues that would not be seen on an x-ray.

Mast cell: A type of immune cell, often found on the surface linings of organs, that is involved in allergic reactions.

Metabolism: The body's building up of new body tissues from food sources and breaking down of those food sources to derive energy. This building up and breaking down, life sustaining process within the body requires the burning of calories and this metabolic rate determines the number of calories burned per hour.

Methotrexate: A powerful drug, with many potential side effects, used in the treatment of rheumatoid arthritis.

Minocycline: A form of the antibiotic tetracycline currently being tested in a clinical trial as a treatment for rheumatoid arthritis.

Monoclonal antibody: A laboratory-replicated antibody being used experimentally to diminish inflammatory reactions in the body.

Myofascial Pain Syndrome: This syndrome describes a localized aria of muscle and surrounding tissue pain and/or tenderness.

Neuritis: Inflammation of nerves.

Nightshade: A botanical family that includes potatoes, eggplants, tomatoes, peppers (red and green bell peppers, chili peppers and paprika). Some people believe the nightshade family can cause joint inflammation.

Nitrates: Food preservatives found in cured meats and some other foods that may cause joint swelling in some people.

Nonsteroidal anti-inflammatory drugs (NSAIDs): A group of drugs having pain-relieving, fever-reducing and anti-inflammatory effects due to their ability to inhibit the synthesis of prostaglandins. Includes aspirin, ibuprofen and many prescription drugs.

Nutritionist: A person who provides nutritional counseling. Although some nutritionists are well trained and knowledgeable, anyone, regardless of training, can call himself a nutritionist.

Occupational therapist: A health-care professional who provides services designed to restore self-care, work and leisure skills of people who have specific performance incapacities.

Omega-3 fatty acids (also called eicosapentaenoic acid, or EPA): Fatty acids found in fish such as mackerel, sardines and salmon, and shown to inhibit inflammation in the body.

Orthopedist (or orthopedic surgeon): A doctor who specializes in surgery of the joints and related structures.

Oscilloscope: An instrument that displays a visual representation of electrical variations on a fluorescent screen.

Osteoarthritis: Degenerative arthritis, often caused by joint injuries or old age. The most common type of arthritis.

Osteonecrosis: Death of bone cells.

Penicillamine: A drug, related to penicillin, that is sometimes used to treat rheumatoid arthritis.

Pericarditis: Inflammation of the pericardium, the fibrous tissue surrounding the heart.

Placebo: A supposedly inert substance, such as a sugar pill or injection of sterile water, that may be given under the guise of effective treatment. In "controlled" clinical research studies, a group of people taking a placebo is compared with a group receiving the treatment being studied. The placebo group is called the "control group." Studies show that about one-third of the people taking a placebo—for any reason—show an improvement in symptoms, at least initially. That phenomenon Is called the "placebo response."

Plaquenil: Brand name for an anti-malaria drug (hydroxy-chloroquine) that is used to treat rheumatoid arthritis.

Platelet: Disk-shaped blood element that tends to adhere to damaged or uneven surfaces and help blood to clot.

Primary-care physician: The doctor you're most likely to see first for most illnesses. May be a general practitioner, a family practitioner or an internist.

Prostaglandin: Hormonelike substance produced in the body from fatty acids. Prostaglandins have a variety of effects, including the control of inflammation.

Psychologist: A nonmedical professional (usually with a Ph.D. in psychology) who may offer various forms of psychotherapy. A psychologist cannot prescribe drugs.

Psychoneuroimmuinology (PNI): A new field of study that is concerned with the mind and how it can affect our immune system's complex network of vessels, internal organs, and white blood cells. The fascinating fact about this field indicates that the vital body systems, the brain and the immune system, communicate through a rich network of blood vessels and influence one another. This field has been created recently by scientists al over the world such as psychiatrists, endocrinologists, neuroscientists, immunologists, and microbiologists that have united their fields of expertise.

Purine: Protein compound, found in anchovies, organ meats, mushrooms and other foods, that can aggravate gout by elevating body levels of uric acid, which crystallizes in joints.

Range-of-motion exercise: Exercise specifically designed to keep a joint flexible.

Registered Dietitian (R.D.): A nutritional counselor who has been certified in dietetics by the American Dietetic Association (ADA).

Remission: Diminution or abatement of the symptoms of a disease.

Revision: An operation to repair or replace an artificial joint that has loosened, broken or become infected.

Rheumatic disease: A condition that involves inflammation and degeneration of connective tissues and related structures. Such diseases can affect the joints, muscles, tendons and ligaments, heart and lungs, skin and eyes, as well as the protective coverings of some internal organs.

Rheumatoid arthritis: A chronic disease with inflammatory changes occurring throughout the body's connective tissues.

Rheumatoid factor: A protein, found in the blood of many people with rheumatoid arthritis, that indicates the presence of inflammation in the body.

Rheumatoid nodule: Small round or oval bump just under the skin found in some people with rheumatoid arthritis.

Rheumatologist: A doctor who specializes in the treatment of arthritis, especially rheumatoid arthritis and other inflammatory diseases.

Sacroiliac joint: The tailbone; five fused vertebrae wedged between the bones of the pelvis.

Scleroderma: A condition that involves thickening of the skin and changes in blood vessels and the immune system.

Solanine: A chemical substance found in plants such as tomatoes and potatoes. In large amounts, solanine may produce joint inflammation.

Splint: A rigid or flexible appliance to immobilize or protect inflamed joints.

Sternum: A plate of bones forming the breastbone.

Steroid drug: Potent drug related to the hormone cortisol, produced by the adrenal glands. Steroid drugs quickly reduce swelling and inflammation, but have possibly serious side effects.

Subchondral bone: Bone found directly under the cartilage of a joint.

Sulfasalazine: A powerful drug used in the treatment of rheumatoid arthritis. In a preliminary study by Dutch researchers, sulfasalazine was found to slow joint destruction in people with early RA.

Symmetrical: Equal in size or shape (of the body or parts of the body); very similar in placement about an axis.

Synovectomy: The cutting out of a synovial membrane of a joint.

Synovial fluid: Fluid secreted by the synovium, the cells lining a joint capsule, which lubricates the joint and helps nourish the cartilage.

Synovial membrane: The cells lining the inside of the joint capsule, which secrete lubricating fluid. In rheumatoid arthritis, the synovial membrane overgrow the joint capsule, invades the cartilage, and begins to secrete biochemicals that can destroy a joint.

Synovium: The synovial membrane. The cells lining the inside of the joint capsule, which secrete lubricating fluid.

Systemic lupus erythematosus (SLE): A chronic, body-wide inflammatory condition that affects the joints, skin, blood, lungs, cardiovascular and nervous systems, and kidneys.

Tendon: A strong band of tissue that connects muscle to bone.

Tendinitis: Inflammation of a tendon.

Transducer: A device that translates one physical quantity, such as pressure or temperature, to an electrical signal.

Triptergium wilfordii (thundervine root): A Chinese herbal remedy for rheumatoid arthritis currently undergoing clinical trials in China.

Ultrasound: A technique in which deep structures of the body are visualized by recording the reflections (echoes) of ultrasonic waves directed into the tissues.

Uric acid crystal: Tiny, needle-shaped particle that forms in a joint when concentrations of uric acid become high, as in gout.

Vasculitis: Inflammation of blood vessels.

Vegan diet: A vegetarian diet that excludes dairy products and eggs.

Visualization: A method of process of thought utilizing the subconscious mind and the imagination to assist in goal achievement, whether it involves family, career, finances, or simply altering positive thinking on a daily basis to enhance the return to health and vitality in one's pursuit of getting well.

BIBLIOGRAPHY

Absorption and Utilization of Amino Acids, Mendel Friedman, ed. U.S. Department of Agriculture, Albany NY vol. I, II, III, CRC Press, Boca Raton, FL, 1989.

Alexander, J. W., B. B. MacMillan, J. D. Stinnett, C. K. Ogle, R. C. Bozian, J. E. Fischer, J. B. Oakes, M J. Morris, and R. Krummel "Beneficial Effects of Aggressive Protein Feeding in Severely Burned Children," *Annals of Surgery* 192: 505, 1980.

Balch, J. F. & Balch, P. A. *Prescription for Nutritional Healing.* New York: Avery Publishing Group, 1990.

Baldessarini, R. J. "Drugs and Treatment of Psychiatric Disorders," In: L. S. Goodman and A. Gilman, eds., *The Pharmacologic Basis of Therapeutics,* 7th ed., New York: MacMillan, 1985.

Bengtsson, A., and M. Bengtsson "Regional Sympathetic Blockade in Primary Fibromyalgia," *Pain* 33: 161, 1988.

Bennett, R. M. "Beyond Fibromyalgia: Ideas on Etiology and Treatment," *Journal of Rheumatology* 16(supple 19): 185, 1989.

Bennett, R. M., et al. "Low Levels of Somatomedin C in Patients with the Fibromyalgia Syndrome: A Possible Link Between Sleep and Muscle Pain," *Arthritis Rheumatology* 35: 1113, 1992.

Boland, E. W. "Psychogenic Rheumatism: The Musculoskeletal Expression of Psychoneurosis," *Annual of Rheumatological Disorders* 6: 195, 1947.

Brooks, P. M. and Day, R. O. "Nonsteroidal Anti-inflammatory Drugs—Differences and Similarities," *The New England Journal of Medicine* 324(24): 1716-1725, June 1991.

Bucci, L. R. "Reversal of Osteoarthritis by Nutritional Intervention." *ACA Journal of Chiropractic* 27(November 1990): 69-72.

Bucci, L. R. *Nutrition Applied to Injury Rehabilitation and Sports Medicine.* Boca Raton, FL: CRC Press, pp. 140-149, 1994.

Buchwald, D., et al. "The Chronic, Active Epstein-Barr Virus Infection Syndrome and Primary Fibromyal-gia," *Arthritis Rheumatology* 30: 1132, 1987.

Calabro, J.J. *Osteoarthritis Diagnosis and Manage-ment,* Ch. 18: "Principals of Drug Therapy." Philadelphia: W. B. Saunders Co., pp. 317-322, 1992.

Campbell, S. M., et al. "Clinical Characteristics of Fibrositis. I. A 'Blinded' Controlled Study of Symptoms and Tender Points," *Arthritis Rheumatology* 26: 817, 1983.

Carper, J. *Stop Aging Now.* 1st ed. New York: Harper Collins Publishers, 1995.

Chase, T. N. and D. L. Murphy "Serotonin and Central Nervous System Function," *Annual Review of Pharmacology* 13: 181, 1973.

Childers, N. F. *Arthritis—A Diet to Stop It: The Nightshades, Aging and Ill Health.* Gainesville, FL: Horticultural Publications, 1986.

Clement, C. D., ed. *Anatomy of the Human Body.* 30th ed. Philadelphia: Lea and Febiger, 1985.

Cousins, Norman. *Anatomy of an Illness: As Perceived by the Patient.* New York, NY: W. W. Norton & Co., 1979.

Cousins, Norman. *The Healing Heart.* New York, NY: W.W. Norton & Co., 1983.

Crofford, L. J. et al. "Hypothalamic-Pituitary-Adrenal Axis Perturbations in Patients with Fibromyalgia," *Arthritis Rheumatology* 37: 1583-1592, 1994.

Dexter, P. and Brandt, K. "Distribution and Predictors of Depressive Symptoms of Osteoarthritis." *Journal of Rheumatology* 21(2): 279-286, 1994.

Dollwet, H. H. A. *The Copper Bracelet and Arthritis.* New York: Vantage Press, 1981.

Dunne, F. J. and C. A. Dunne "Fibromyalgia Syndrome and Psychiatric Disorder," *British Journal of Hospital Medicine* 54: 194-197, 1995.

Elrod, J. M. *The Body Advantage: Total Wellness System.* Montgomery, AL: Dr. Joe M. Elrod and Associates, 1996.

Elrod, J. M. "How Not To Be a Dropout," Newsletter, *Sportrooms of America,* Vol. 3: 27, 1982.

Ferraccioli, G. F. et al. "EMG Biofeedback in Fibromyalgia Syndrome," *Journal of Rheumatology* 16: 1013, 1989.

Fischbach, F. A. *Manual of Laboratory Diagnostic Tests.* 3rd ed. Philadelphia: J. B. Lippincott, 1991.

Gans, D. A. "Sucrose and Delinquent Behavior: Coincidence or Consequence?" *Critical Reviews in Food Science and Nutrition* 30(1): 23-48, 1991.

Garnett, L. R. "Strong Medicine," *Harvard Health Letter,* pp. 4-6, 1995.

Gay, G. "Another Side Effect of NSAIDs," *Journal of the American*

Medical Association 264(20): 2677-2678, November 28, 1990.

Germaine, B. F., M.D. "Silicone Breast Implants and Rheumatic Disease," *Bulletin on the Rheumatic Diseases* 41(October 1991): 1-4.

Gold, P. W., M.D. "Stress Response and the Regulation of Inflammatory Disease." *Annals of Internal Medicine* 117 (November 15, 1992): 854-66.

Gowers, W. R. "Lumbago—Its Lessons and Analogues," *British Medical Journal* 1: 117, 1904.

Goldenberg, D. L. et al. "A Randomized Controlled Trial of Amitriptyline and Naproxen in the Treatment of Patients with Fibromyalgia," *Arthritis Rheumatology* 29: 1371, 1986.

Goldenberg, D. L. "Psychological Symptoms and Psychiatric Diagnosis in Patients with Fibromyalgia," *Journal of Rheumatology* 16(suppl 19): 127, 1989.

Goldenberg, D. L. "Fibromyalgia and Chronic Fatigue Syndrome: Are They the Same?" *Journal of Musculoskeletal Medicine* 7: 19, 1990.

Goldenberg, D. L. et al. "High Frequency of Fibromyalgia in Patients with Chronic Fatigue Seen in a Primary Care Practice," *Arthritis Rheumatology* 33: 1132, 1990.

Goldenberg, D. L. et al. "The Impact of Cognitive-Behavioral Therapy on Fibromyalgia," *Arthritis Rheumatology* 34(suppl 9): S190, 1991.

Goldenberg, D. L. "Fibromyalgia: Treatment Programs," *Journal of Musculoskeletal Pain* 1(3/4): 71, 1993.

Goldenberg, D. et al. "A Randomized, Double-Blind Crossover Trial of Fluoxetine and Amitriptyline in the Treatment of Fibromyalgia," *Arthritis Rheumatology* 39: 1852, 1996.

Granges, G. and G. Littlejohn "Prevalence of Myofascial Pain Syndrome in Fibromyalgia Syndrome and Regional Pain Syndrome: A Comparative Study," *Journal of Musculoskeletal Pain* 1(2):19, 1993.

Hauri, P. and D. R. Hawkins "Alpha-Delta Sleep," *Electroenceph Clin Neurophysiology* 34:233, 1973.

Hendler, N. and Kolodny, A. L. "Using Medication Wisely in Chronic Pain," *Patient Care*, 6:125-139, May, 1992.

Hendler, S. S., M.D. *The Doctor's Vitamin and Mineral Encyclopedia.* New York: Simon and Schuster, 1990.

Hess, E. V., M.D. and A. Mongey, M.D. "Drug-Related Lupus," *Bulletin on the Rheumatic Diseases* 40(August 1991): 1-7.

Hobson, J. A. "Sleep After Exercise," *Science* 162: 1503, 1968.

Hodgkinson, R. and Woolf, D. "A Five Year Clinical Trial of

Indomethacin in Osteoarthritis of the Hip Joint." *ACTA Orhtop Scand.* [AU: PLS. Confirm] 50: 169, 1979.

Jaeschke, R. et al. "Clinical Usefulness of Amitriptyline in Fibromyalgia: The Results of 23 N-of-1 Randomized, Controlled Trials," *Journal of Rheumatology* 18: 447-451, 1991.

Kelley, W., M.D., et al. *Textbook of Rheumatology.* Philadelphia: W. B. Saunders, 1989.

Lehninger, A. L. *Biochemistry,* The John Hopkins University School of Medicine, Worth Publishers, Inc., Sixth Edition, NY, 1972.

Mankin, H. J. *Arthritis Surgery: Clinical Features of Osteoarthritis.* Philadelphia: W. B. Saunders Co., pp. 469-479, 1994.

May, K. P. et al. "Sleep Apnea in Male Patients with the Fibromyalgia Syndrome," *American Journal of Medicine* 94:505,1993.

McCain, G. A. et al. "A Controlled Study of the Effects of a Supervised Cardiovascular Fitness Training Program on Manifestations of Primary Fibromyal-gia," *Arthritis Rheumatology* 31: 1135, 1988.

McCarty, D. J., M.D. *Arthritis and Allied Conditions: A Textbook of Rheumatology.* 11th ed. Philadelpha: lea and Febiger, 1989.

Miller, B., M.D., and C. B. Keane, R.N. *Encyclopedia and Dictionary of Medicine, Nursing and Allied Health.* 4th ed. Philadelphia: W. B. Saunders, 1987.

Moldofsky, H. D. et al. "Musculoskeletal Symptoms and Non-REM Sleep Disturbance in Patients with 'Fibrositis Syndrome' and Healthy Subjects," *Psychosomatic Medicine* 37:341, 1975.

Moldofsky, H. D. "A Chronobiologic Theory of Fibromyalgia," *Journal of Musculoskeletal Pain* 1(3/4): 49, 1993.

Moldofsky, H. D. "Sleep, Neuroimmune and Neuroendocrine Functions in Fibromyalgia and Chronic Fatigue Syndrome," *Advances in Neuroimmunology* 5:39-56, 1995.

National Research Council. *Recommended Dietary Allowances,* p. 1, Academy of Sciences, Washington, DC, 1980.

Novak, K. K., et al. *Drug Facts and Comparisons.* St. Louis, MO: Facts and Comparisons, Inc., 1995.

Nxrregaard, J. et al. "A Randomized Controlled Trial of Citalopram in the Treatment of Fibromyalgia," *Pain* 61: 445-9, 1995.

Panush, R. S., M.D., ed. *Rheumatic Disease Clinics of North America: Nutrition and Rheumatic Diseases.* 17(May 1991). Philadelphia: W. B. Saunders.

Panush, R. S., M.D. "Food-Induced ('Allergic') Arthritis: Inflammatory Arthritis Exacerbated by Milk" *Arthritis and*

Rheumatism (February 1986) 220-6.

Panush, R. S., M.D. "Food Induced ('Allergic') Arthritis: Clinical and Serologic Studies." *Journal of Rheumatology* 17(No. 3, 1990); 291-4.

Pellegrino, M. J. et al. "Familial Occurrence of Primary Fibromyalgia," *Arch Phys Med Rehabilitation* 70: 61, 1989.

Pisetsky, D., M.D. *The Duke University Medical Center Book of Arthritis.* New York: Fawcett Columbine, 1991.

Quillin, P. "The Role of Nutrition in Cancer Treatment," *Health Councilor* 4(6).

Quillin, P. *Healing Nutrients,* Contemporary Books, Inc., Chicago, IL, 1987.

Rooney, T. and Rooney, P. *The Arthritis Handbook.* New York: Balantine Books, 1986.

Russell, I. J. et al. "Treatment of Primary Fibrositis/Fibromyalgia Syndrome with Ibuprofen and Alprazolam—A Double-blind, Placebo-Controlled Study," Arthritis Rheumatology 34:552, 1991.

Russell, I. J. et al. "Elevated Cerebrospinal Fluid Levels of Substance P in Patients with the Fibromyalgia Syndrome," Arthritis Rheumatology 37:1593-1601, 1994.

Russell, I. J. "Neurochemical Pathogenesis of Fibromyalgia Syndrome," Journal of Musculoskeletal Pain 4:61-92, 1996.

Sandler, D. P. "Analgesic Use and Chronic Renal Disease," The New England Journal of Medicine 320:1238-1243, 1989.

Saskin, P. et al. "Sleep and Post-traumatic Rheumatic Pain Modulation Disorder (Fibrositis Syndrome)," Psychosomatic Medicine 48:319, 1986.

Schroder, H. D. et al. "Muscle Biopsy in Fibromyalgia," Journal of Musculoskeletal Pain 1(3/4):165, 1993.

Schumacher, H. R., M.D., ed. Primer on the Rheumatic Diseases 9th ed. Atlanta: The Arthritis Foundation, 1988.

Sciarillo, W. G. "Lead Exposure and Child Behavior." American Journal of Public Health 82(10):1356-1359, 1992.

Sheon, R. P., M.D., et al. Coping With Arthritis. New York: McGraw-Hill, 1987.

Simms, R. W. et al. "Lack of Association Between Fibromyalgia Syndrome and Abnormalities in Muscle Energy Metabolism," Arthritis Rheumatology 37:801-807, 1994.

Simonton, O. et al. Getting Well Again. 3rd ed. New York: Bantam Books, 1992.

Simonton, O. and Simonton, S. "Belief Systems and Management of the Emotional Aspects of Malignancy." Journal of Transpersonal Psychology 7(1):29-47, 1975.

Smythe, H. "Fibrositis Syndrome: A Historical Perspective," Journal of Rheumatology 16(supple 19):2, 1989.

Sobel, D., and A. C. Klein. Arthritis: What Works. New York: St. Martin's Press, 1989.

Stehlin, D. "How to Take Your Medicine—Nonsteroidal Anti-inflammatory Drugs." FDA Consumer pp. 33-34, June 1990.

Stinnett, J. D. Proteins and Amino Acids-Prospects for Nutritional Therapy in Infection, In Relevance of Nutrition to Sepsis, Ed. J. E. Fischer, Ross Laboratories, Columbia, OH, 1982.

Tenney, L. The Encyclopedia of Natural Remedies, 1st ed. Woodland Publishing Co., Pleasant Grove, UT, 1995.

"The 5-A-Day Easy Eating Plan," The Johns Hopkins Medical Letter, 5(2), April 1993.

U.S. Department of Health, Education, and Welfare, Healthy People, 101, U.S. Government Printing Office, 79-55071, Washington, DC, 1979.

Theodosakis, J., Adderly, B., and Fox, B. The Arthritis Cure, Ch. 5: "The Problem with Pain Killers," New York: St. Martin's Press, pp. 69-80, 1997.

Vestergaard-Poulsen, P. et al. "31P NMR Spectroscopy and Electromyography During Exercise and Recovery in Patients with Fibromyalgia," Journal of Rheumatology 22:1544-1551, 1995.

Wallace, D. J. et al. "Fibromyalgia, Cytokines, Fatigue Syndromes, and Immune Regulation," In: Advances in pain Research and Therapy, J. R. Fricton and E. Awad, eds., Raven Press, v. 17:227-287, 1990.

Weil, A., M.D. Natural Health, Natural Medicine. Boston: Houghton Mifflin, 1990.

Weintraub, S. Natural Treatments for ADD and Hyperactivity. Pleasant Grove, UT: Woodland Publishing, 1997.

Werbach, M. Nutritional Influences on Illness. Tarzana, CA: Third Line Press, 1988.

White, K. P. et al. "Work Disability Evaluation and the Fibromyalgia Syndrome," Semin Arthritis Rheumatology 24:371-381, 1995.

Wolfe, F. "Fibromyalgia: The Clinical Syndrome," Rheumatology Dis Clin North America 15:1, 1989.

Wolfe F. et al. "The American College of Rheumatology 1990 Criteria for the Classification of   Fibromyalgia: Report   of   the

Multicenter Criteria Committee," *Arthritis Rheumatology* 33: 160, 1990.

Wolfe, F. "Fibromyalgia: On Diagnosis and Certainty," Journal of Musculoskeletal Pain 1(3/4): 17, 1993.

Wolfe, F. "The Epidemiology of Fibromyalgia," Journal of Musculoskeletal Pain 1(3/4): 137, 1993.

Wolfe, F. et al. "A Double-blind Placebo Controlled Trial of Fluoxetine in Fibromyalgia," Scandinavian Journal of Rheumatology 23(5): 255-9, 1994.

Yunus, M. B. et al. "A Controlled Study of Primary Fibromyalgia Syndrome: Clinical Features and Association with Other Functional Syndromes," Journal of Rheumatology 16(supple 19):62, 1989.

Yunus, M. B. et al. "Relationship of Clinical Features with Psychological Status in Primary Fibromyalgia," Arthritis Rheumatology 34(1):15-21, 1991.

Resource List

The Fibromyalgia Network
P.O. Box 31750
Tucson, AZ 85751-1750
800-853-2929 or FAX 520-290-5550.

The American Fibromyalgia Syndrome Association, Inc.
6380 E Tanque Verde Rd. Ste. D,
Tucson, AZ 85715
520-733-1570

Fibromyalgia Association of Central Ohio
P.O. Box 21988
Columbus OH 43221-0988
614-457-4222

American Association for Chronic Fatigue Syndrome
7 Van Buren Street
Albany, NY 12206
518-482-2202

Fibromyalgia Association of Greater Washington, Inc.
12210 Fairfax Towne Center, Ste. 500
Fairfax, VA 22033
703-790-2324

Fibromyalgia Association of Texas
3810 Keele Dr.
Garland, TX 75041
214-271-5085

Inland Northwest Fibromyalgia Assoc.
9209 E. Mission, Ste. B
Spokane, WA 99206
509-921-7741

Fibromyalgia Times
P.O. Box 20408

Columbus, OH 43221-0990
614-457-4222

Fibromyalgia Frontiers
P.O. Box 2373
Centreville, OH 22020
703-912-1727

Arthritis Foundation
P.O. Box 19000
Atlanta, GA 30326
800-283-7800

Fibromyalgia Educational Systems
500 Bushaway Road
Wayzata, MN 55391
612-473-6218 or 419-843-3153

The CFIDS Association of America, Inc.
P.O. Box 220398
Charlotte, NC 28222-0398
800-442-3437

Massachusetts CFIDS Association
808 Main Street
Waltham, MA 02154
617-893-4415

Restless Legs Syndrome Foundation, Inc.
304 Glenwood Ave.
Raleigh, NC 27603-1455
919-834-0821

Seattle Fibromyalgia International Team, Inc.
P.O. Box 77373
Seattle, WA 98177
206-362-2310

The TMJ Association
6418 W. Washington Blvd.

Milwaukee, WI 53213
414-259-3223

Fibromyalgia Association of BC
Box 15455
Vancouver, BC V6B 5B2 Canada
604-430-6643
The Ontario Fibromyalgia Association
250 Bloor Street, E. Ste. 901
Toronto, ON V4W 3P2 Canada

The Arthritis Society, BC Division
805 West 10th Avenue
Vancouver, BC V5Z 1L7 Canada
604-879-7511

American Association for Marriage and Family Therapy
1133 15th St. NW, Ste. 300
Washington, DC 20005
800-374-2638

American Psychiatric Association, APA
Department AT, 1400 K St. NW
Washington DC 20005
202-682-6220

American Psychological Association
750 First St. NE
Washington, DC 20002
800-374-3120

Depression, Awareness, Recognition and Treatment (D/ART)
5600 Fishcers Lane, Rm. 10-85
Rockville, MD 20857
800-421-4211

National Alliance for the Mentally Ill
200 N. Bleve Rd., Ste. 1015
Arlington, VA 22203-3754
800-950-6264

National Association of Social Workers
750 First St. NE, Ste. 700
Washington, DC 20002
202-408-8600

National Depressive and Manic Depressive Association
730 N. Franklin, Ste. 501
Chicago, IL 60610
800-82N-DMDA or 800-826-3632

National Foundation for Depressive Illlness
P.O. Box 2257
New York, NY 10116
800-248-4344

National Mental Health Association
1021 Prince St.
Alexandria, VA 22314-2971
800-969-6642

American Academy of Allergy and Immunology
611 E. Wells St.
Milwaukee, WI 53202
414-272-6071

American Academy of Environmental Medicine
P.O. Box 16105
Denver, CO 80216
303-622-9755

American Apitherapy Society
P.O. Box 74
North Hartland, VT 05052
802-295-8764

American Association of Acupuncture and Oriental Medicine
4101 Lake Boone Tr., Ste. 201
Raleigh, NC 27607
919-787-5181

American College of Rheumatology
60 Executive Park S., Ste. 150
Atlanta, GA 30329
404-633-3777

American Dietetic Association
430 N. Michigan Ave.
Chicago, IL 60611

American Holistic Medical Association
2002 Eastlake Ave. E.
Seattle, WA 98102
206-322-6842
American Nutritionists Association
P.O. Box 34030
Bethesda, MD 20817

Ankylosing Spondylitis Association
511 N. LaCienega Blvd., Ste. 216
Los Angeles, CA 90048
800-777-8189
310-652-0609 (in California)

Arthritis Foundation
1314 Spring St. NW
Atlanta, GA 30309
800-283-7800

Food Allergy Network
4744 Holly Ave.
Fairfax, VA 22030-5647
703-691-3179

Lupus Foundation of America
4 Research Pl., Ste. 180
Rockville, MD 20850-3226
800-558-0121

National Chronic Pain Outreach Association
7979 Old Georgetown Rd., Ste. 100

Bethesda, MD 20814
301-652-4948

National Commission for the Certification of Acupuncturists
1424 16th St. NW, Ste. 501
Washington, DC 20036
202-232-1404

National Institute of Arthritis and Musculoskeletal and Skin Diseases
NIH Information Clearinghouse
Box AMS
8000 Rockville Pike
Bethesda, MD 20892
301-495-4484

National Institute of Arthritis and Musculoskeletal and Skin Diseases
Multipurpose Centers

Middle Atlantic

Cornell University Medical College
The Hospital for Special Surgery
Research Building, Room 605
535 East 70th St.
New York, NY 10021
212-606-1189

Midwest

Case Western Reserve University
2074 Abington Rd.
Cleveland, OH 44106
216-844-3168

Indiana University School of Medicine
541 Clinical Dr., Room 492
Indianapolis, IN 46202-5103
317-274-4225

Northwestern University Medical School
303 E. Chicago Ave., Ward 3-315

Chicago, IL 60611
313-503-8197

New England

Brigham and Women's Hospital
75 Francis St.
Boston, MA 02115
617-732-5356

Boston University School of Medicine
71 E. Concord St., K5
Boston, MA 02118
617-638-4310

University of Connecticut School of Medicine
263 Farmington Ave.
Farmington, CT 06030-1310
203-679-3605

Pacific

Stanford University
100 Welch Rd., Ste. 203
Pal Alto, CA 94304

University of California, San Diego
Department of Medicine, 0945
La Jolla, CA 92093
619-558-1291

University of California, San Francisco
P.O. Box 0868
San Francisco, CA 94143-0868
415-750-2104

University of California School of Medicine
10833 LeConte Ave., 47-139 CHS
Los Angeles, CA 90024-1736
213-825-7991

South

University of Alabama at Birmingham
UAB Station, THT 429A
Birmingham, AL 35294
205-934-5306

University of North Carolina at Chapel Hill
932 FLOB, UNC-CH School of Medicine
Chapel Hill, NC 27514
919-966-4191

AUDIO/VIDEO AND OTHER MATERIALS

Fibromyalgia: One Day Seminar (1993/1994): Audio tapes of day-long forums sponsored by the Arthritis Foundation Rocky Mountain Chapter. Includes sessions by rheumatologists, neurologists, psychiatrists, psychologists, and occupational therapists. To order: Arthritis Foundation, Rock Mountain Chapter, 2280 South Albion St., Denver, CO 80222-4906, 303/756-8622 or call 800/475-6447 for an order blank. Website: http://www.arthritis.org. Cost: $6 each or $5 each for three or more.

What's New in Fibromyalgia–Third National Seminar (1994): Series of seven videos and 16 audiotapes about basic research, growth hormone factors, exercise, long-term outcomes, post-traumatic fibromyalgia, legal issues, coping with fibromyalgia, and a "ask the experts." Some information too technical for average audience, although much useful information is covered. For more information contact Fibromyalgia Alliance of America, P.O. Box 21990, Columbus, OH 43221-0990, 614/457-4222. Cost: $30 per video or $165 for complete set of seven videos; $15 for set of two audiotapes for $75 for complete set of 13.

The Body Advantage (1996), by Dr. Joe M. Elrod: Elastic stretch exercise device including video with complete exercise program designed specifically for fibromyalgia and arthritic sufferers. To order: Call 334/272-3605 or write to 3074 Zelda Road, Suite 190, Montgomery, AL 36106

Aspirin and Other NSAIDs (1996): This 16-page brochure discusses aspirin and other nonsteroidal anti-inflammatory drugs, including dosage, side effects, and important tips to remember when taking them. To order one copy: Arthritis Foundation, 1330 W. Peachtree St., Atlanta, GA 30309, 800/283-7800. To order copies in multiples of 50: P.O. Box 6996, Alpharetta, GA 30329,

800/207-8633.

Coping with Depression in A Chronic Illness (1995): This 14-page brochure is a helpful primer on coping with and accepting change. To order: Michigan Lupus Foundation, 26202 Harper Ave., St. Clair Shores, MI 48081, 810/775-8310. Cost: $3.50 plus $1.50 shipping/handling.

The Drug Guide (1995): Originally featured in the July/ August issue of Arthritis Today, this 10-page guide will educate you about the drugs you take for your arthritis. To order one copy: Arthritis Foundation, 1330 W. Peachtree St., Atlanta, GA 30309, 800/283-7800. To order copies in multiples of 50: P.O. Box 6996, Alpharetta, GA 30329, 800/207-8633.

Mid-Atlantic Conference on Fibromyalgia Treatment (1996): Proceeding of the September 1996 conference are available on audio cassette. Set of six 90-minute Audio cassettes. To order: Fibromyalgia Association of Greater Washington, D.C. (FMAGW), Suite 500, 12210 Fairfax Towne Center, Fairfax, VA 22033, 703/790-2324. Cost $72 for general public.

The Success Journal, Elrod, Dr. Joe M. Montgomery, AL: kinner Printing/Dr. Joe M. Elrod & Associates, 1996. To order: Call 334/272-3605 or write to 3074 Zelda Road, Suite 190,. Montgomery, AL 36106.

To contact Dr. Elrod regarding consultation, speaking engagements, or for other further information, use the following information:

Dr. Joe M. Elrod
3074 Zelda Rd. Suite 190
Montgomery, Alabama 36106
phone: (334) 272-3605
fax: (334) 279-3117

INDEX